ANDALUCIA

For Gayle , Andy
and your beautiful children
with love and thanks
– Richard x

PRAISE FOR KICKED OUT

A novel to stand up alongside Irvine Welsh's Trainspotting, offering a window into the youth of today. A fantastic book expressing the cynicism and dissatisfaction of those on the edge of society

Waterstone's Recommended Read

The narrative is so strong, the characters and dialogue so real, the situation so heart-breaking. This is masterful and should win several literary prizes

Patricia J. Delois, author of Bufflehead Sisters

Hardwick's writing has the power and humanity to make you wonder about the way you see the world, and to give voice to those whose stories usually remain untold

Laura Brewis, New Writing North

A truly compelling page-turner

Inside Time, the National Newspaper for Prisoners

Hard-hitting, at times hilarious...fantastic

The Crack

ANDALUCIA

RICHARD W HARDWICK

LAPWING
BOOKS

Lapwing Books

31 Southward

Seaton Sluice

Northumberland NE26 4DQ

ISBN 978 - 0 - 9569555 - 0 - 0

Cover by Tustin Design

Printed and bound in Great Britain by Martins The Printers in
Berwick-upon-Tweed

For Anna, Joe and Isla…

PART I

She's on her feet before her surname echoes off the wall behind. Towards the smiling nurse she strides. I get up slower, gather my book, my empty bottle of water, shuffle after. But then I'm spotted. And the nurse takes her gaze from Anna's slim face, her long brown hair. And her expression changes as her hand comes up.

"She's only going for the..."

Mumbles something like she doesn't want to say the words.

I presume Anna's going to sign her name, check details, will be back in two minutes. Surely I'll be allowed to support her all the way through? So I wander back across the waiting room, look round at faces that fall away rather than make eye contact. And I sit back down in Anna's chair, still warm. The door does open two minutes later but it's the nurse that comes out. I sling her a dirty look, turn to the telly, watch history unfolding. Barrack Obama smiles back at me. Helicopter pictures of the celebrating masses. Braving the weather, that's what the presenter says. While around me, in warm silence, sit ten or so people; waiting to hear about themselves or their loved ones.

Inauguration:

To commence officially or formally; to initiate.

The doctor had said, "It doesn't feel like cancer," smiled affectionately. Anna returned the smile and then the nurse smiled too. I remembered to breathe out again. Everything's going to be alright; that's what all the smiles meant.

"But you need to have the mammogram," he added. "Just in case"

And I'm still here. And it's getting on for an hour now. And I couldn't give a toss that the world might be changing for the better. Eventually she comes out, slower than she went in, a little unsteady on her feet, says they had to test some cells. They'd squished her this way and that. It was bigger than it seemed. They have to stick a needle into it, send it to the lab. I hold her hand, still warm and inviting; grip it tighter than I normally would.

Then we're back in the same room as before and the doctor pushes a long thin needle into her breast and the tears come rolling down her cheeks as she grits her teeth against the pain. And the nurse holds her shaking hand while I sit uselessly at the foot of the bed.

"Pretty worried," is what the doctor says this time. "That's why they have the mammogram, the ultrasound. It's difficult to tell just from feeling"

And then more waiting. Except this time we've moved along the conveyor belt and the silence has a thickness that's rarely challenged. Now there's just six, the lucky ones allowed to leave, take their relief with them, return to normal lives. A woman's legs buckle. She's picked off the floor and taken to a private room. The doctor rushes in. An hour later a nurse pushes her out in a wheelchair, past legs that move quickly, eyes averted elsewhere. Two more go in and then come out, just a quick five minutes for both of them. And then, second from last, after two more hours of waiting, two more hours of hand holding and leg rubbing, they call out her name again...

This time we go past the room we've already been in three times, the room we've seen others go in, come out of. Two doors down is where we go. A different nurse introduces herself, says the doctor will be along in a few minutes.

And we sit there. And we look around at the leaflets on the wall. And we know...

Cancer is your name. But many call you Big C.

It's shorter. And easier.

Thirty-six years old with cancer. A girl that people always turn to when things fall apart. A girl that always knows the right thing to do, the right thing to say.

But she can't answer the question the nurse asks her.

"Do you have any children?"

She breaks down and I answer instead. Explain we have a five year old boy called Joe. A two year old girl called Isla.

9

She asked if she had the right group, seemed a little nervous, sat down on carpet and crossed legs, black hat perched above dyed black hair, black clothes flowing all around. After a few seconds studying carpet pattern she looked up and across at the four blondes in designer clothes lined up on the chairs. Then she glanced at my flowery shirt, my slicked back pony tail, and she felt very different. And though it wasn't love at first sight for me either, I'd be lying if I said I wasn't interested.

She sat next to Pete on the aeroplane, swapped with Helen because he was terrified of flying, held his hand while we took off. Over Western and Eastern Europe we went, out over the Mediterranean, round the south of Turkey and above Cyprus until eventually Tel Aviv slipped into sight down below. There was nothing political in my choice of destination. I'm not Jewish and I wasn't going to work with oppressed Palestinians. I was simply going as far away from London as I could with what money I had, away from ecstasy and the dull blur of alcohol, away from the office job that was never as exciting as people pretended it was. I was twenty-one years old, going to work the land, sweep clean my mind. I was going for an adventure. And if love came around too; well, that would be a bonus. Anna was eighteen, had three months before starting nursing training. She wanted to go to Nepal with a lad she fancied, sold everything she had in a car boot sale but didn't make enough money so joined the Sheffield kibbutz group instead. But they didn't fly for another month and she wanted to leave straight away. The London group agreed to take her but needed to check availability, then quickly responded with the news that there was just one seat left on the plane. Anna got it.

On such small details whole lives and families are created.

A large cemetery came into focus as we descended, tiny rectangles of gravestones in orderly rows, trees greener than those in England, streets and fields drier, white buildings illuminated in a land used to fierce sun. Over a busy dual carriageway and down to a runway and a round of applause that brought bemused looks from nine young Brits. Past the suspicious questions of customs, the furrowed brows of armed soldiers, through a dark alley with railings on either side, staring people crushed outside, arms and legs flailing through. And into a waiting minibus.

The driver didn't speak much, just straightened his gun on the dashboard, pressed down on accelerator. I sat next to Anna as we bounced on hard seats, looked out at wide streets, people drinking coffee outside cafes, white and pale modern buildings, military camps with high walls. Leaving the city behind, we journeyed through camel coloured fields, past clusters of houses as seen on TV, hitch-hiking soldiers and ancient gnarled trees. Shirley passed forward a Motown tape. Giggles turned to song. The driver looked in his mirror and smirked. Past Jenin and through Afula we went, round the southern tip of the Sea of Galilee as the last of the sun fell away behind us. Then, the tape finished, we drove up, up, up into the darkness of the Golan Heights. Aware we were on occupied territory the minibus fell into apprehensive silence as we started to wonder about our destination; Kibbutz Afiq. The woman at Kibbutz Representatives explained it was the nearest settlement to both Jordan and Syria, saw our concerned faces and said, 'Don't worry, there's an army regiment based there the whole time.' Eventually we reached the top and continued over flat land and what seemed like nothing else until we sighted small lights on our right beyond high barbed wire fences. The driver slowed. And we pulled up at large gates in front of a manned and armed watchtower, highlighted by our headlights in the darkness.

~

I push the trolley down the aisle looking for cooking chocolate. I push back the tears as well, as some cliché ridden pop song plays softly over the speakers, a song I would have ignored two days earlier, probably mocked.

She wants to stay positive she says, as we walk down the beach hand in hand.

I leave her at six thirty a.m. to drive to work, leave her for the first time since the news, leave her with both children because Joe has a temperature, is too unwell to go to school. I feel guilty but she wants everything to be as normal as possible, and anyway we need the money. And if I don't go to work, I don't get paid. I can't focus; just stand there while everyone else makes small talk. Those that know why I was off two days ago come up and then push back their own tears while I find myself reassuring them. We're not thinking worst case scenario I say. It doesn't bear thinking about. It slips in now and then but we shove it back out, slam the door shut. And then I cross my fingers and hope the same is true of Anna back home.

Sometimes I get a feeling in my stomach like a cramp that folds over, that twists tighter and tighter, squeezes nausea upwards like bile through internal tubes. I eat my breakfast and chat to oblivious children. I don't ask what Anna gets. Then I telephone my Mam. I've been putting it off. When someone's on the vulnerable and rocky road to recovery themselves, and they don't know if they have the energy, then it's the last thing they need. The phone's engaged. She'll be on the Internet looking for inspiration, searching for techniques. Googling medication.

I've nearly finished the seventh pint before I can bring myself to do it, before a quiet moment allows. It's not an easy thing to just slip into conversation. We're outside The Free Trade pub, looking down at the Tyne, the Baltic, the Sage, the Millennium Bridge. They've been at our house all day and they haven't got a clue. I wanted to tell them over the first pint, give it time to settle. But they were so happy, the atmosphere so good. We don't meet up that often these days. One shrugs in drunken sympathy, declares she'll get through it. The second says nothing, just listens, then talks about something personal he's been through. The third freezes in all but eyes, unable to speak, rooted into paralysis as he remembers a past family member. I take another sip and apologise for not telling them earlier.

Everyone's gone. The kids are in bed. She's outside looking at the stars as the tears slowly roll. It's harder at night-time, away from children that think everything's normal, away from work and its distractions. We cuddle but I can't think of anything to say that hasn't been said a dozen times already. I tell her I love her once again, make sure I don't cry with her. I have to be a rock; that's what people say. I can crumble into pieces when she's not present. But I have to be solid when she's nearby.

It lays further down, in the unconscious, smothering everything else. Dominating. It's been pushed down there but tiny droplets seep out. This isn't a tap that can be fully turned off, perhaps ever. Music is its gateway, or at least it is this time. It seems wrong to be driving to work, to be driving away from her, but we need the money and she's at work herself for the time being. I tire of Radio 4's company, the aid to Gaza advert, the reclassification of cannabis (again), the scandal of corrupt politicians (again). So I put a CD on. It starts gentle enough but when the guitars kick in I feel the first signs of movement inside tear ducts. I feel my foot pressing harder on the accelerator, picture myself driving wildly. Then I picture myself on stage, smashing my guitar, smashing my fist into someone's face. And then finally I picture myself at home in the kitchen, smashing my fists off cupboards, throwing things off the shelf, destroying the place. I pull into the prison car park surprised to have arrived in one piece and completely unaware of the last half hour's drive. Perhaps my unconscious is not completely smothered after all.

Six-twenty a.m. and I'm downstairs in the kitchen making sandwiches. I hear Anna asking Joe to go to the bathroom and get washed and dressed. Joe growls, stamps his feet like a baby elephant, shakes the ceiling above me. Anna plays things exactly the same way she always does; calm yet firm. But Joe screams at his Mammy and so I shout upstairs. Anna tells me she's dealing with it, go walk the dog. I leave the house and wonder how I would cope on my own, how I would manage to get everything done. I wonder how a five year old boy and almost three year old girl, both of whom adore their Mammy, would cope with her death; whether their beautiful, funny, self-absorbed little minds would crack like eggs. Or fill like dirty sponges. And I let a few tears slide down because I can. I'm on my own, and it's still dark.

~

"Straight out the gates. Keep going. Turn right at the dead cow"

We were off to find the ancient ruined city of Piq, following directions we got from three nervous German girls we met at the volunteer houses. We never saw the cow, walked out over flat dusty land, the occasional green rectangle of orchard sighted in the distance. We stood on a deserted road, watched the sun set deep orange over mountains that could have belonged to Israel, Syria or Jordan for all we knew then. And then we turned back to Afiq, our new home.

All the girls except Anna and Helen were still downbeat about our accommodation. Jane physically gasped when we arrived at them. Although ours were the same as all the rest from the outside; small, white, single story and very basic, the inside gave a new meaning to minimalism. One living room with a couple of tatty couches, a shower room with toilet and three bedrooms with nothing except thin mattresses on low metal frames. Be sure to shut the doors we were told. And don't leave windows open. Jane was disgusted. This wasn't what she expected; Sarah, Sharon and Shirley too. They were after parties, hedonistic fun, at the very least a few posters on the walls. Nobody had alcohol either. Everyone stupidly thought there'd be a shop open more than two afternoons a week. We stayed up late chatting, discovering each other, met Marla in the morning, the American volunteer co-ordinator. Our first day was free. The day after we'd be working in the gardens and would have to wear strong boots because five dogs had been killed by snakes that summer.

We arrived back from our unsuccessful quest to find Piq, found the swimming pool instead, had a dip as the dark thickened. The German girls came along, still seemed hesitant, eventually said there'd been problems with English volunteers in the past. They often didn't stay because life was too simple, work too hard. Afiq had only been a kibbutz since 1972, was the first Israeli settlement established in the Golan Heights after the Six Day War, was small and isolated compared to most other kibbutz. And if English volunteers did stay they drank too much to alleviate the boredom. The last group had just left, were lazy, got drunk every night. One lad drove the tractor into the swimming pool pissed. If we wanted respect and friendship in a place like this we would have to earn it. Rob and I walked to the phone box on the other side of the kibbutz to reassure worried mothers, sidestepped a black scorpion, hurdled a cockroach being attacked by hundreds of ants and noticed on the outside of the perimeter fence, a deer being chased by what looked like wild dogs.

The tide is out, the clouds are parting and the air is crisp; a perfect January day. Halfway along the beach I see a hunched figure coming towards me, stick in hand; someone who already knows. Minutes later, Brian stands and faces me.

"Well, it's a beautiful day isn't it?"

I nod, shrug...

We watch our dogs a moment. Then he moves alongside me and we look at the sea. And he asks how Anna is.

He nods as I talk. He's "been there, got the t-shirt." And all he has now are memories and photographs he can't look at. He tells me people used to come up when he was walking the dog and ask how his wife was. He felt like punching them he said, had to remind himself it was only because they cared. But if he saw them coming towards him, even if it was close enough for them to see him, he used to turn away, walk in a different direction so they wouldn't meet.

He needs to move on before I do.

I carry on down the beach, looking for shells and stones to take back home. Down by the waves I walk, tip-toeing like a sandpiper, using the approaching roar as my retreat signal. Moving fast when white foam crashes at my feet. I scan them, thousands, millions even, some flesh coloured, stretched sinews and tendons. Others dappled like horses. Speckled thrushes. They're better where the waves come. The water brings out their colour, their energy, highlights and contrasts. And then something catches my eye, lodges in my gut at the same time. Part of an animal perhaps. Sea creature cut out with rough knife. I stand above it and look down in disgust. Nodules stick out, tubes clogged wet with sand. I'm fascinated and revolted at the same time, want to pick it up and examine it, throw it far into the sea. But I can't bear to touch it, so I kick it instead. It's hard like bone. I kick it into the flush of the waves and continue along the beach without looking back.

The full moon illuminates fields and rolling hills, soft with overnight snow. It pulls me to work, not away from it. I don't understand and then I realise it's because it's my last day for a week and a half. I want to get to work so I can get back again. I turn left, just five minutes away and now the moon tries to pull me home. It wouldn't make any difference. It's Anna's last day too, probably for months. Her operation is in two days time. I remember how she couldn't sleep. I took her a cup of tea in the early hours of the morning. She laid on her side and repeated the same thing.

"I just want to come back. I just want to come back"

Out we staggered, through purple sunrise to strong coffees, rakes and hoes after two hours sleep. By noon we'd spent seven hours clearing weeds and dried grass. Then, as we ate dinner of boiled chicken, rice, stale bread and salad, and pretended not to be bothered by the feast of eyes upon us, we watched them come up the stairs one by one. Dark skinned, short black hair underneath hats pulled down tight, dark blue overalls, old green army jackets, sturdy black boots and machine guns slung over shoulders like any other accessory. The Golani, the army regiment stationed at Afiq, came up for dinner and looked us all up and down, but in particular the girls.

On the night we found the disco, an underground bomb shelter invisible from the air. Gingerly down dark steps we went, but Israeli Goldstar beer was good, better than the music. So we got drunk and watched Golani dance around machine guns like handbags. Then Anna and I drank black coffee and went to Piq with Yasmin, one of the German girls. We sat on top of bombed Syrian houses destroyed in the 1967 war, built on ancient ruins from centuries before. Looked down the valley as the sun rose golden over Tiberius and the Sea of Galilee. The sky above shifted slowly from black to grey, white to pale to deep blue; the valley from murky brown to burnt orange like faded memories from Sunday School. Hyrax, known as rock rabbits, popped heads out of holes one or two at a time until there were dozens on either side, sunning themselves on rocks. Birds sang praises and the Galilee sparkled and shimmered like there really was divine creation.

PART II

It starts just like any other day. Anna's drying her hair and I'm trying to get Isla's tights on while she stamps her feet up and down. And Joe hasn't uttered a single word to anyone because he's too busy saving the world in his bedroom. Then the taxi comes and Anna's kissing and hugging and in far too much of a rush to get emotional. Two and a half hours later the kids are on their way to school and child-minder. And by half ten I've ticked everything off Anna's list and I'm kicking my heels against wooden floorboards. It's unlikely I'll be able to see her until six p.m. but I can't stay this far away, have an increasing need to be near her. I drive through falling snow to the metro station, leave my car in an illegal spot and pass a traffic warden on the way in. I'm allowed forty minutes with her. I hold her hand; watch her take clothes off, put robes on, Paris Hilton white stockings. She's quiet, seems somehow reflective, even before the event. I wonder how she manages to do it; stay so calm, so graceful. And then she's led away and I follow. The nurse says we can kiss but she'd rather we didn't do tongues. And then Anna walks away from me, steps into the lift and doesn't turn around. I stand and watch the doors close, the orange light move down through the numbers. Then turn away.

I'm sipping hot coffee, eating an almond muffin, listening to some David Gray-a-like strum and moan. I'm staring out the window, watching people desperately try and keep their feet in back street slush. Anna will be unconscious, under the knife. I remember the pre-assessment two days ago; best case scenario lump removed, followed by radiotherapy for a few weeks and a return to normal life. I remember looking around the waiting room at anxious faces, nobody talking, just the occasional subdued whisper. One teenager, four girls in their thirties, a couple in their fifties; mothers, daughters, wives, girlfriends, workmates, best friends, neighbours. And then I looked at Anna. And I don't know the statistics, I'm completely ignorant. But I looked around the room again. And I thought at least one of you is going to deteriorate rapidly and die very soon. And I'm nervous, so nervous, that it's going to be Anna.

I'm by her side now, holding her hand. The pain's contained, medicated. It's her stomach she's worried about. She hasn't eaten for twenty-four hours, says she's starving but they won't let her eat. Her breast has swollen. They think she has a haematoma, that the wound has started to fill up with blood. They'll let her come home tomorrow but she might need to go back in, have further surgery. We hold hands but don't talk. And inside we pray that this is the end of it all.

Her shout comes directly through the ceiling above me.

"Can you come upstairs please?"

She's been in the shower. Maybe she wants help getting dried, can't reach her back. But I go upstairs and there she is, crouching on the bathroom floor naked, holding a flannel to her breast. Blood trickling down her stomach, three blood-soaked flannels by her feet. I get the first aid kit out, tell her it's just nature's way of sorting things out, taking away swelling, easing the tension. In truth I don't have a clue. She holds the flannel a few more minutes whilst I wipe blood away from her stomach, her legs, the floor. She takes it away five times but the blood keeps seeping out. I wash the garlic and salt off my hands and open a sterile dressing.

We're on the bathroom floor again, but this time it's three in the morning. The dressing's soaked through dark red and the blood's seeping out. The door is shut so children can't see the light, don't come and investigate. I take the dressing off slowly while Anna gets ready to catch any flowing blood. She dabs as it comes out, while I remark how her breast looks much more natural now the bruising has gone, how it's almost returned to normal size. Anna is as calm as usual. The pressure has reduced and with it the pain. Things are returning to normal. We smile at each other and tip-toe back to the bedroom hand in hand, confident about results later today.

At the noise of approaching engine, we jumped up with enthusiasm, five of us stood in a line. Pushed our arms out and stuck our thumbs down as advised. The car went straight past, left nothing but rising dust in the distance like some seventies western. Half an hour later the next car came and we repeated the same movement like some amateur bedraggled dance troupe; Pete with his shorts and t-shirt sleeves rolled up, his moustache and balding head, Helen with her long legs and long blonde hair, Anna with her flowing skirt and skimpy vest top, me with my painted Doctor Marten boots and football top and Rob with his skinny freckled Scottish legs. And so, perhaps understandably, the second car went past too. We'd decided to hitch-hike after being told it was normal practice, and Shabbat was our only day off each week. Out through the gates we'd gone, into the flat dusty vastness of the Heights, a few green bushes sprouting here and there amid a 360 degree horizon of sun scorched grass and earth. We'd followed the track from Afiq until we reached the one road that came out there, headed for the shade of the bus-stop, an isolated sanctuary from heat riddled with bullet holes. And then someone else came along; a soldier from Afiq. He smiled but carried on straight past, stood about twenty metres further down. A car came along just a few minutes later. Again we performed what was fast becoming a natural manoeuvre. Our spirits lifted as the car slowed down, then sank as it went right past us and picked the soldier up, who got in without looking back. After another failed attempt and the realisation that a bus hadn't been past in the last hour and a half either, we decided on an astute tactical move. We sat back in the shade, supped from water bottles, then when we heard the next car only Anna and Helen stepped out. This time the car slowed down, right to a stop, and one of the girls held the door open for Rob, Pete and I to climb in. Along the top we went, then down in slow curls, riding camel coloured earth waves frozen in motion, rising and peaking, ebbing away before rising and peaking once more. And then we were right down, almost seven hundred feet below sea level, at the lowest freshwater lake on earth, following palm trees along the shore of the Galilee where Jesus recruited disciples from local fishermen. We were dropped off at En Gev, a rich kibbutz hidden behind trees, then walked down its side to the water's edge where the son of God told numerous parables and performed many miracles. Over volcanic and limestone rock, to millions upon millions of tiny shells embedded in thick dry mud to form a beach. The water was bottle green, warm as a welcome bath, breathing slowly. We waded out, dipped our bodies in, looked at hills and valleys that surrounded us, white painted Tiberius on the far side. Anna, Helen and I fell asleep near where the tide softly broke, woke up with water lapping around our bodies. Then, feeling blessed, we hitched a lift within minutes with a middle aged bearded man. He took a different route, pulled his car into the side about three quarters of the way up. We followed him to a viewing site, sat on a low wall and looked out at the whole of the Sea of Galilee, hazy in the heat like our sun stroked minds, fed on the right by the Jordan River that ran down between Syria and Lebanon.

Our driver waited patiently for us to take it all in, then held his arm out, swept it along.

"Do you know where you are?" he asked rhetorically. "The Sea of Galilee with the miracles of Jesus. And the city of Tiberius, named after the Roman Emperor. Destroyed by two earthquakes"

He reminded us we were standing on Syrian earth, where they bombed Israel from before it was captured in 1967.

"You can see why this is so necessary for Israel," he said, sweeping his hand backwards, motioning to the whole of the Golan. "If you are down there, you have no chance"

We walked back to the car in silence, wondering if he was Israeli or Arabic. Then he drove us back to the top, along the road to Afiq and dropped us off right outside the gates.

Anna lies on the bed whilst the nurse changes her dressing and comments how nature does indeed take its course. The breast looks almost as it did originally, bar a small concave area and an obvious incision mark where they cut into it. I smile, remember the teenage lad on the metro opposite, all intrigued when she pulled her top out and peered downwards to see if the dressing was doing its job. The nurse disappears. Anna unfolds her newspaper, reads the two front page headlines; a genetic master switch which would allow cancer to be turned off. And how Jade Goody's children will live with their father when she dies.

Then the doctor comes in.

He brings another nurse with him, a medical student too. Opens the file with eyes cast down. Looks up and tells us her results. The invasive cancerous lump was small and has been removed successfully. But when they opened her up there were pre-cancerous cells around it that hadn't been detected. Also, two of the four lymph nodes they took out of her armpit were infected with cancer. They have no option but to remove the whole breast, to start a course of chemotherapy and radiotherapy, to prescribe Tamoxifen and probably Herceptin too. They'll also have to take more lymph nodes out, probably all of them, because it's through these that cancer spreads, if it hasn't already. I look at Anna, mouth on hand. Stunned. The doctor looks at us both in sympathy. But we can't speak so he says a little more. The medical student fidgets, doesn't know where to put herself. And still we can't speak. And so the doctor asks if we understand everything. Anna nods, clamps her knuckles with her teeth at the same time, understands perfectly. It's everything we didn't want to hear. She's going back for surgery. The cancer may have spread through her body. She's going to have her breast cut off, have chemotherapy every three weeks for six months. Her hair is going to fall out. And there's a chance that the cancer will kill her, will kill Joe and Isla's Mammy. As usual, she thinks little of herself and more of how they would cope. The doctor leaves and her head goes down. And the tears flow out. The student squirms and slips away. The nurse gives us a few minutes alone. I try my best to fight back tears but eventually break and join her.

Days of work followed. I partnered an Israeli called Rufel, climbed ladders, cleared ivy from gutters and roofing. Anna cleared grass with Helen and a few others. On the afternoon we sat outside our houses in the sunshine, wrote letters and diaries, walked to Piq or the Syrian House on the other side of kibbutz, watched kaleidoscope sunsets down valleys and over the Galilee; always Anna, Helen, Rob and myself. I watched Anna and Helen move whenever I could, like I watched them move in the waters of the Galilee. I watched them come back from work together, chat and laugh, become great friends.

Out walking in the Golan, we came across an old Howitzer, its long barrel pointing down at dusty earth; then nothing, no landmark at all except the odd withered tree. Until half a mile later, a half destroyed bus. Further on, an old desert coloured army truck. We took pictures of ourselves in them like excited children, idiot tourists brought up in a peace taken for granted. We found pillboxes and trenches along the top edge of the Golan that spied down on Tiberius and the Galilee. Crawling through them we discovered rusty beds burrowed inside rock, tried to imagine what this alternative reality must have been like. The next evening Rob and I ventured out the kibbutz in the dark, to a phone box by the side of the road, using light from thousands of stars as our guides. The haunting cries of wolves echoed around us like wailing ghosts of Syrians destroyed in the fight for their homeland. We hurried to the safety of the phone box, stood inside during each other's calls. On the way back two of them walked alongside us, just far enough back on the edge of our sight for us to make out the faint silhouettes of their bodies. Howls came from the other side of the road, out in the darkness, thirty, forty feet away. But these two walked silently alongside, as if leading us back to where humans belonged, back inside the tall wire fences of Afiq.

Joe's a tall five year old, slim built with hair in between wavy and curly, in between finally turning from blond to brown. People look at Anna and I, both brunettes, then ask where Joe gets his blond locks from. I tell them he looks like the fruit and veg man who used to come round every Thursday in his shiny new van; that Anna was always quick to climb his little steps, caress his cauliflowers. And he certainly took a shine to Anna as well; of that there's no doubt. Those who know us well laugh my suggestion off easier. They see not only my height and sometimes languid style in Joe, but other characteristics too. The way he completely ignores everything you say if his mind is somewhere else, even if your face is right in front of his. The way he can't see any point in putting effort into something he isn't interested in. And in his otherworldliness and his love of books.

Isla is a different kettle of fish, blessed with beauty like her brother but with lips that can turn from smile to pout and back again within seconds, all framed by long straight brown hair. And if you put your face inches from hers and sharply insist she did something you'd likely be heading for a slap. Joe can be bribed. Threats and treats usually work, especially if they're related to something he values, like pudding or telly or books. Isla will stare and stamp her feet. She'll call your bluff or make a pre-emptive strike. If she doesn't get books until she's brushed her teeth then so be it; she'll just go straight to bed instead. And she'll do it with a swagger rather than a stomp. Her favourite hobby is changing her mind. And her favourite word is "actually."

Disgruntled at having one bottle of wine between eleven at the Shabbat meal, Anna, Rob and I waited until everyone had left, then sneaked though the kitchens and stole seven unfinished bottles. At the time we felt little shame in this. After all, one opened bottle of wine was placed on every table and most Israelis drank very little. It wouldn't keep for a whole week until the next Shabbat surely? However, like naughty children getting away with something and enjoying the rewards, this soon developed into a weekly habit, much to the amusement of the Golani. They came over to our table quite often, sometimes even ventured up to the far edge of the kibbutz where our volunteer houses were situated. Sharon, Shirley and Helen had been along to their section of houses, nicknamed The Bronx by the rest of the kibbutz. Of course the soldiers were more interested in females than males, and the girls didn't seem to mind. Attention from swarthy young males with machine guns, with an underlying sensitivity too, captured in a situation beyond their control, inspired notions of romance and excitement. There were female soldiers too, and it always seemed odd to see girls younger than me, hair down their backs, carrying Uzi submachine guns. But they were content to stay within their group in the main, not venture out our way. With the exception of Marla and Denis, her American footballer husband who converted to Judaism to raise a family in the Golan, and a couple of others, the residents of Afiq said very little to us, just nodded or smiled or did neither. The soldiers though; they worked with us, were away from their homes too. About thirty in number, they were separated into eighteen year olds who had just joined the army and would soon have to see 'real' service, and those in their early twenties who were finishing their final year and were up at Afiq to recuperate before going home. They saw young people their same age, from another side of the world, and they looked at us in wonder, sometimes in envy. To be brought up in peace, to be free of paranoia as you walked down the street, to not have to worry about invasion of your country or being called upon to invade another, to be able to roam the earth and discover new worlds. This was all something they found difficult to comprehend.

My first day back at work. I walk alongside huge concrete walls, damp lichen curling over the top, climbing out from inside, rising from the bottom too, as if reaching out fingers to help. What look like barnacles crust into the middle, standing their ground. Fixed into position to keep the two growths apart. The singing of birds in nearby trees is disturbed by the barking of guard dogs stretching their vocal chords, straining at the leash. I walk into the staff entrance, take my shoes and belt off. Empty my pockets.

People want to know how the results went, expect good news. I've decided five is the maximum number of people I can speak to. I wanted to go out for dinner, get away from everyone, but there's a leaving buffet. I'm eating crunchy bread and paté when someone slides up to me.

"Alright? Where have you been then? Off on holiday?"

He nearly spits his pork pie out when I tell him. Two minutes later, another colleague tells me dogs can smell cancer; start behaving differently. I feel blank in response, can't think of anything to say. Can't remember our dog acting any different.

We plan to spend the day in the garden, sorting out a timetable for the coming six months, how to get the vegetable plots bursting with goodness. But I need to send out invites for the launch of my first novel and Isla is off nursery sick and needs attention. So the day becomes a couple of hours instead. It's Anna's favourite place, the garden. Under these circumstances it could prove the difference between life and death. I pull old sprout plants out, cut them into the compost, tell myself I need to pull my weight in the garden more, research cancer and the immune system.

Joe's watching Teenage Mutant Ninja Turtles, climbing onto the arm of the couch and jumping off, seeing how far he can propel himself through the air before landing on the wooden floor. And all this without taking his eyes off the telly. Another text comes through, one of many, the same as phone calls. Anna replies to most of the texts, leaves the majority of phone calls unanswered. Says she can only manage one conversation a day. If she answered the phone every time, accepted all requests to pop round, she'd be talking about her own cancer from the moment she woke up to the moment she put her head down. I pick the Sunday paper up, see the headline, "Cancer deaths to double in next forty years," put it down instead, turn the radio on to find football scores, find out Eastenders Wendy Richard died just hours ago from the same disease.

Walking Caffrey early morning I see Brian about fifty metres away, stick in air, border collie ready to spring into action. I turn left instead, head away from him, towards the dene and muddy puddles. He doesn't see me. But I'm sure he'd understand.

I get a group e-mail from Richard, Anna's brother, about the annual summer party weekend he throws. He updates everyone on his wife's pregnancy, then tells about Anna, states "survival has been downgraded from very good to good." The sentence sticks in my throat, highlights stark truth, no matter how positive I want to be. It sounds terrifying. I don't see the larger percentage that makes up 'good' when I read that sentence. I see the removal of 'very.' I see the smaller percentage, the one that stands for death, the one that's increased, that could still be growing. My brother-in-law works just a few corridors away from where Anna was diagnosed. He's a doctor.

My sister phones, the first time I've spoken to her since Anna was diagnosed with cancer. She breaks down on the phone, eventually gets it together again, says she loves us all, will do anything she can to help. I'm on the Internet, researching. Anna doesn't want to herself, says she'll take advice from me but won't alter her lifestyle too much. I don't understand. Her basic knowledge is far greater than mine. I have to start from scratch. But maybe that's part of the reason. I read how chemotherapy and radiotherapy destroy healthy cells as well as cancerous ones, how they do more harm than good according to some reports, how some people recommend going nowhere near them. I read that a study of more than six hundred cancer patients who died within thirty days of receiving treatment showed chemotherapy probably caused or hastened death in twenty-seven percent of cases. In only thirty-five percent of these cases was care judged to have been good by the inquiry's advisors, with forty-nine percent having room for improvement and eight per cent receiving less than satisfactory care. I read a study that shows chemotherapy can change the blood flow and metabolism of the brain in ways that can linger for ten years or more after treatment, that this could help explain the confusion, sometimes called "chemo brain," reported by many chemotherapy patients. And The Times' website tells me 300,000 patients now receive chemotherapy in the UK each year, a sixty per cent increase compared to 2004. Furthermore, cancer causes thirteen percent of all human deaths. And according to the American Cancer Society, 7.6 million people throughout the world died from cancer during 2007. I don't tell Anna about these findings. She'll put her life in the hands of the medical profession. She comes from a medical background. It's the only thing she can do. If there's any complimentary medicine or vitamins on offer and the medical profession don't argue against them, then she'll have those too she says, as long as there aren't too many.

I come up with four supplements that are said to be vital in fighting cancer, but then I find another four, and then more too. We can't afford all of them and Anna won't pop loads of pills each meal time anyway. I don't know which ones to buy. I don't know which would be more useful, which could be vital. So I click on four, close my eyes and hope for the best.

We bounced along on the back of a trailer, half asleep and holding on for dear life as the sunrise slowly announced itself and smoke from our cheap cigarettes curled upwards to meet it. Fifteen minutes later a large man with curly black hair and straight face introduced himself as Amit, showed us a square of wood with a circle cut out the middle. We were picking apples he said, and he didn't expect any that fitted through the circle. They were too small and had to be left on the trees. We set off in pairs, apple measurers around necks on string, four empty buckets each. When we filled our buckets they had to be emptied into large crates which were moved by tractor to ensure they were always in front of us. The picking was hard work and by seven in the morning the sun started to burn. But it was soothing too, once you got used to the boss barking instructions, as it took so little concentration, allowed your thoughts to wander. I worked with Rob down one line of trees while Anna and Helen had the next. Amit followed, checked trees, shouted we'd missed apples. Then he went and checked crates and shouted we'd put apples in that were too small. It was not a joke he said. The future of kibbutzim depended upon agriculture. The fruit went all over Israel, some of it abroad too. It was the kibbutz's main source of income. They couldn't survive without it. At eight we were back in the cabin eating omelette and salad for breakfast, speaking quietly as Israelis shouted across the table in Hebrew. Then we were given water bottles and sent back to work. I wandered along with Rob, climbed trees, chatted, found comfort in the combination of activity and silence. Whenever the opportunity arose though, my gaze drifted backwards to the two English girls smiling and chatting their way through the line of trees next to us. Faster they went, driven by childish competition that didn't want boys to finish in front of them. I smiled and pointed, told them they'd missed some, would be in trouble. We stopped for cigarette breaks when the boss wasn't around, sat crossed legged on the earth. That's when I first became aware of Anna and myself staring into each other's eyes, losing ourselves in a whirl of iris, in wonder and admiration. But there were times when we couldn't look each other in the eye, when we had to look away, had to look anywhere but the eyes. I knew during those early days which way my hopes were turning. But there was one significant stumbling block. Anna was returning to England in December to study to be a nurse. Helen, like me, had no timescales to adhere to.

We're on a wild manure hunt armed with wellies, spades and empty bags. After an hour we find some by the side of the road, a large pungent heap beautifully ready. We decide we should ask at the farm but the gate's padlocked so we just help ourselves instead, all of us getting stuck in. As I dig out the better manure from the bottom of the pile, the top caves in and a little field mouse jumps comically for its life and scampers away. We fill eight bags and put them in the boot, then go home for dinner. Then we go to the school field for bike practice, assault course and family football. Nobody talks about cancer, about life or death. We simply live for the moment. And it's a beautiful day, a perfect Sunday.

It's last thing at night before bedtime. She's in the shower when she notices this one as well. She doesn't shout me upstairs, just waits until I walk into the bathroom, says it matter of fact. Points to her other breast.

"I've got another lump"

I move forwards, press my finger into her breast and squash it, just above the nipple. It's there alright. It doesn't feel much, just a tiny firm lump the size of a pea, a little smaller than the one on the other breast but similar in all other ways. It moves when I press it, like it's trying to evade me singling it out, slip back to being unnoticed until it can spread its vile malignance further. Anna stands there in some kind of daze, water dripping from her naked body.

"It might not be cancer," I say. "You'll probably think it is just because of the last one, but it might not be"

She doesn't look at me.

"It feels like the last one," she says.

"Yeah I know, but the last one felt like a cyst according to the doctor so that's no definite sign"

She smiles. One of those flat ones

"And even if it is, then it's probably better to find it now anyway. Better that than wait two years down the line and think you're in the clear"

Her face does nothing so I continue mumbling whatever comes into my head.

"They can probably just deal with everything in one go as well"

And then she looks up at me, scared puppy dog eyes.

"But can they operate on both at the same time?"

"I don't know," I admit. "I don't know"

And I reach out to her naked body and pull her in close.

I'm going for lunch with Kathleen, a colleague and friend who's been through it all herself fourteen years ago. She takes my hand, tells me everything will be alright, looks at me with eyes that understand. I telephone Anna who starts crying on the phone. The hospital doesn't have any appointments until Thursday and that's with a nurse, not a doctor, so she can't be examined. She's waiting for our GP to phone back, needs to speak to someone today. Needs someone to tell her that there really is a lump in her other breast. That she's not imagining it.

"There is," I say. "I felt it"

"I know," she says. "But I need to see someone today. I need to speak to someone"

"I'll cancel my class this afternoon, come back home"

"No, don't worry"

"It's not a problem. Everyone's really understanding here"

"Honestly. It's okay. Helen's coming round in her lunch break. I'll be fine, really I will"

So I put the phone down because she's waiting for the doctor to ring. And Kathleen smiles gently, tells me everything will be alright.

We go for a walk across the cliffs, just the two of us and Caffrey. We walk right along the edge, look down at waves and rocks, curlews and gulls. Remember the time we saw what looked like the body of a shark washed up. When we first moved here I used to cycle along these cliffs to sign on in Whitley Bay, then sit down on an overhanging rock and write, wait for Anna coming back from work. It's the first time she's been here for years. It's not the place to take young children, right on the edge, and it's me who does the early morning and late night dog walking. We hold hands all the way, reminisce further; how we used to clamber over rocks together, take hours because we had no responsibilities, no time constraints. We look for the giant hole where we joked King Rabbit must have lived. Remember how we used to see men with guns and dogs out hunting. Hawks perched on shoulders. You don't see hunters out here anymore. Disease has wiped most of the rabbits out.

The Golani came round most nights after a week or two; names like Hagai, Itsic, Moses, Uzi, Yossi and Hanan. It was a mutual fascination between us and them, outsiders together but a world apart in every other sense. Hesitant at first, they dropped by in groups of two or three. They asked about England, about London, hoped they would be able to travel themselves when they left the army. The older Golani said little about their military experience, found mutual interests and pressed these instead. Did we like The Doors? Velvet Underground? The Beatles and the Stones? Simon and Garfunkel? We made a fire, played chess, drank cheap Russian vodka from Tiberius. I played my tapes: Primal Scream, Van Morrison, KLF, Neil Young. A passing German called Holgar told of a place on the edge of the Egyptian Sinai Desert called Dahab. Said people of all nationalities went there to smoke cannabis, take opium, listen to Hendrix and Marley, scuba dive and chill by the sea. I added it to my agenda, straight in at the top of the list. He told us about Jerusalem, said we had to visit, but that two German girls were murdered there a few days before for being western. It happened in the Arab quarter where he told us to go to a cafe and ask for water pipe and hash. In the meantime, I climbed down rocks from Piq, found a fresh spring, picked fruit from the pomegranate tree, brought them back for Anna who was feeling off colour. Then one night, fed up with not being able to buy beer and sometimes cigarettes at the shop because kibbutz residents and soldiers were allowed in before volunteers, we set off at half past ten to walk to Bnei Yehuda, a settlement with a shop and pub more than a mile away. Three English and one Scot, walking through the Golan Heights in the pitch black, shuddering at the howling of wolves. Motivated by alcohol rather than adventure. On the way back, we laid down flat on the road. Looked up at a sky full to bursting with stars, pin pricks in heaven. Watched meteors enter the earth's atmosphere, streak above us, leave behind shining trails of gas. Then, after just a few hours sleep, we were up again, spending the morning in baking heat, on cherry picking machines that allowed us to zoom up to the larger apple trees with our buckets. Anna, Helen and I agreed on a cigarette break every hour. Wherever we were in the orchards, we pulled the lever down until we rose higher than the trees, could see mile upon mile of Golan, watch the colour of the sky change, look out for eagles and vultures, wave to each other, lean back carefully and enjoy our smoke.

On the next Shabbat, Anna, Rob, Pete and I decided to hitch-hike to Hamat Gader on the Jordanian border. After walking for three hours in boiling heat we split into pairs to see if it made things easier. All the boys wanted to go with Anna. The company of a pretty girl was motivation enough but it also meant you were more likely to get picked up. Rob won. So he and Anna got a lift before Pete and I, who had to wait another half hour and then were dropped off a mile before our destination and had to walk along the road by the barbed wire and electric border fence. We were stopped three times by soldiers, advised to turn back at the border post of watchtowers, jeeps, Howitzers and rocket launchers. Still, on we continued. Anna and Rob were waiting at the gates with nervous smiles. Being Afiq volunteers we were able to get in without paying, due to some arrangement with the kibbutz that probably included free avocados, apples or chickens. We stripped off and sampled the bubbling hot water, fed by mineral rich hot springs that welled up from deep underground. Then we walked around the ruins, tried to imagine two thousand years before, when it was one of the largest and most luxurious health resorts in the Roman Empire. Finally, the alligator farm and a picnic on the grass, where we looked up from our low position to the two mountains either side of us, one Israeli occupied, the other Jordanian. And then, as our eyes returned towards ground level, we noticed for the first time, soldiers with machine guns on the roof of the expensive restaurant.

Cancer is a mistake cell that is growing wildly out of control, that may consume the patient through malnutrition, organ failure or infection. Nearly all cancers are caused by abnormalities in the genetic material of transformed cells. These abnormalities may be due to the effects of carcinogens such as tobacco smoke, radiation, chemicals, or infectious agents. Other cancer-promoting genetic abnormalities may be randomly acquired through errors in DNA replication, or are inherited, and thus present in all cells from birth.

On such tiny details whole lives and families can be ripped apart.

Primary causes of cancer include:

◆   Poor nutrition; leading to an excess, deficiency or imbalance of certain nutrients

I put the book down and stare out the window. Anna has a better diet than anyone I know. She loves fruit and vegetables, salads and seafood, hardly ever eats fatty foods or ready meals. In the garden last year she grew potatoes, spinach, kale, carrots, broccoli, beans, peas, radishes, turnips, beetroot, tomatoes, cucumbers, chillies, peppers, watercress and about five different types of lettuce. I walk into the kitchen, open a cupboard door. These are the different types of herbal teas we've got: revitalise, detoxify, clarity, peppermint, chamomile and spearmint, nettle, fennel, ginger, green tea, white tea, Egyptian spice, perk me up and sleep easy. Anna likes all of them. Combined they alleviate insomnia, relax nerves, relieve anxiety, reduce fever, reduce pain and swelling, eliminate excess fluids, enhance weight loss by reducing appetite, lower cholesterol, prevent tooth decay; soothe stomach aches, allay ulcers, bladders, kidneys and urinary tract ailments, cleanse the colon, soothe and promote healing of minor burns and skin irritations, provide the essential elements and dietary minerals lacking in our bodies, protect us from the formation of free radicals by neutralizing them before they can cause cellular damage and disease, promote endurance, increase stamina, enhance memory, improve circulation, boost the immune system, act as a digestive aid for nausea, vomiting and motion sickness and ease irritable bowel syndrome and menstrual cramps. I shake my head, shut the cupboard and walk back to my book to find out the second primary cause:

♦ Stress; the mind generates chemicals that can lower protective mechanisms against cancer

Anna is the most stable person I know, the most stable person I have ever known. People have always come to her when they're in need of balance and neutrality, when they require a safe haven of calming energy, someone to listen without judgement. I feel like throwing the book through the window. This isn't the way things were supposed to be. This wasn't Anna's role in life, just like it wasn't her mother's and her mother's before that. She comes from a female blood line of angels upon earth. She's had one day off sick in the last seven years. She's never been a victim in her life.

♦ Sedentary lifestyle; exercise helps to oxygenate and regulate the entire body

The only programme Anna sits down and watches is Gardeners World; that's half an hour a week. And she often doesn't read until she's lying in bed. She cooks, cleans, washes, chases after children, digs, plants and walks the dog. Since moving up to the North East nine years ago she's worked on the home care, walking round the village looking after the elderly, then taken people with physical and learning disabilities out into their communities. Before that she worked as a massage therapist, massaging people with terminal cancer, and for the home care service in London. She doesn't sit at a desk, fiddling around on a computer or answering the telephone. She couldn't.

♦   Toxic burden; hence detoxification becomes crucial

I look to my mother, her allergies in this unnatural world we've created through our desire for progress, power and money, our fascination for technology and our need to fit into a world that gets faster and faster. I wonder about all the fruit and vegetables we've eaten, the chemicals that have been sprayed upon them to stop nature taking place, disease or pests consuming profits. If you took all the pesticides we've eaten throughout our lives, added them together and then offered the collection to us to drink right now, would there be a glassful or a bucketful? I think of the time Anna worked as a cleaner, squeezing out bleach, oven cleaner, multi surface sprays and bathroom mousses, ironically all with fragrances such as lavender, pine and lemon fresh; how she tried not to breathe in or had to leave the room for half an hour because of the fumes. And all those times when she just had to get on with it, breathe the fumes because she had to get finished on time. Had someone's ironing to do before they came back from this slavery trap of modern life. And I wonder....

The dark had set in hours before. We carried on because there seemed no other choice. Pete was in a good mood, whistling and making up limericks. And he walked behind

Anna and I most of the way, which was fine by us. Our initial intention was to walk all the way round the Sea of Galilee but we'd set off too late, probably for the best as we hadn't realised it was more than fifty-three kilometres in circumference. Instead we bussed fourteen kilometres to Tiberius with the intention of hitch-hiking from there to Capernaum, where the apostles Peter, Andrew, James and John were born and where Jesus first began to preach to the masses. After half an hour Jane moaned enough for Helen to go back with her, leaving just Pete, Anna and I. By five p.m. we gave up the idea of hitch-hiking in favour of walking as far round the Sea of Galilee as we could, before sleeping in a bus stop until a bus arrived. By six p.m. it was pitch black and we were already tired, just Pete's whistling and silly songs to motivate us. But on we went, because there was nothing else to do. At nine p.m. we reached a fish restaurant next to the ruins of Capernaum and stopped for one beer each, an extravagance we'd earned but could ill afford. Relaxing in welcome light for a change we were approached by a slight English lad called Ricky who described himself as an "alcoholic skinhead from Stoke" and had a tattoo on his forearm spelling 'Riot.' Ricky had been thrown off his kibbutz but had found work at this restaurant during the day. We finished our beers and he walked outside with us, said he was pleased to meet some English people for a change. Off the road we went, along the shore a little, found ourselves a spot. He gave us free beer and wine, steak with pitta bread, ice cream for pudding. We got drunk under the stars, cooked on a fire that lasted all night through, dipped our toes in the Galilee and laughed at Pete, who had a cardboard box to curl up in and looked downright miserable. Anna, Ricky and I settled down on thin mattresses and warmed ourselves to sleep by the fire. Then promising to visit again, we said goodbye to Ricky in the morning and got a hitch straight away, missing completely the new church built on the site of Saint Peter's house, the ruins of the old Roman town, one of the oldest synagogues in the world and an excavated fishing boat from the time of Jesus. Another lift took us to the bottom of the Golan, where Pete accepted a lift to Bnei Yehuda. Anna and I decided to walk. And it was here, among the golden slopes of the Golan, pausing to look back down at the shimmering Galilee with aching legs, that I first realised I was falling in love with the girl beside me. We didn't speak much, just smiled at each other and continued climbing, turned round to convince ourselves we were really there. I touched the top of her sun darkened back, her shoulder that glistened with sweat. I pretended to pull her up, an excuse to hold her hand while she laughed along, and Ricky got the sack back down below. It took us three hours to arrive at the top, another hour to make our way back to Afiq. But there, climbing that dusty road under deep blue skies, unable to venture off track because of signs that warned of landmines, we were as happy as we ever could be.

Anna goes off to Newcastle for her hastily arranged appointment with a breast care nurse, hoping to find something for Isla's birthday beforehand. I pick Joe up from school, ask if he wants a story CD for the car as we're going to get Isla from nursery.

He wants "rock-star" music, asks if I have any.

"Of course." I walk over to my music collection. "I've got lots"

"Yes Daddy, but does it have guitars?"

"Oh yes"

"And drums as well? Does it have drums?"

I smile to myself. This is the moment I've been waiting for. He didn't like "noisy" music before. He preferred classical.

"All rock-star music has guitars and drums Joe"

Fifteen minutes later we're driving through North Shields listening to The Ramones on high volume and I find myself disappointed that Joe isn't trying to jump out of his booster seat, that he hasn't commented how cool the police siren start to Psycho Therapy is. Isla's overjoyed to see her big brother, rushes to cuddle him. I stand there, proud parent of two beautiful, intelligent and sensitive children. Things are different on the way home though. If Isla isn't shouting then Joe's moaning. And if Joe isn't moaning then Isla's shouting. Most of the time though, there's both shouting and moaning. When they start hitting each other I lose my temper, yell at them to behave and keep quiet. But then we turn into our street and Joe spots Anna out the window. His moaning stops instantly and I haven't applied the handbrake before he's running down the street towards her. Isla's not far behind, screaming in delight. I look down the pavement at them all hugging, seatbelt tight to my chest, stopping my heart from falling out. I don't know whether to laugh or cry. They don't have a clue about what's to come, about what their Mammy has to go through, about how it could kill her.

Anna's been reassured by the nurse but can't remember anything she was told. Later she remembers the nurse has worked in breast care for over eleven years and only once has seen cancer spread from one breast to the other. In all other instances of two breasts being infected they've been separate cases of cancer. We look at each other, smile weakly. Every time we've received news so far it's been terrible, the situation worsening. People say 'don't worry, she's young and healthy, she'll fight it off.' I've heard it numerous times. Don't they realise? When you're younger your cells multiply faster. Cancer spreads quicker. But then, what did I know about cancer, even just a few days ago? Since diagnosis she's received mountains of cakes and chocolates from friends, all well-meaning and given with love. Tumours feed on sugars, devour them. It's the worst possible thing you can eat. I look at her; that lost expression when the children aren't around, when she's not doing something to take her mind from it. She's slim, small chested too. It wouldn't have far to travel from one to the other. But I say something designed to be reassuring. She has another appointment on Tuesday, to see if she has cancer in the other breast. And, I presume, to ask about the likelihood of cancer elsewhere; and chances of survival. Tuesday is important for another reason too. It's March 10th; Isla's third birthday.

We were told to stay in the living room with the lights off until the military exercise was finished. A neighbouring kibbutz's soldiers were going to invade and see if they could

47

take over some of the houses. If we'd known what was to happen the very next night we wouldn't have found it all so exciting, wouldn't have smiled at the irony of such timing. The operation was over the other side of Afiq so we couldn't see anything. Instead, we lit a candle and told ghost stories. It only took twenty minutes but nobody told us. We stayed like that for over two hours until someone saw Hagai wandering about. Then, with lights on, we talked about travelling. Anna said she couldn't. It didn't matter how much she wanted to. She had to move to Newcastle in January to start nursing training. Everything was organised. Helen said everyone was getting itchy feet because three weeks had elapsed and with it came the growing realisation that this was not a holiday. We'd signed up for the kibbutz way of life for three months though it was becoming obvious some wouldn't make it that far. Natural groups had formed; me with Anna, Rob and Helen; Sharon with Shirley, Jane with Sarah and Pete by himself. Late at night Anna and I walked across the Golan to the pub at Bnei Yehuda, just the two of us. On the way back we walked beneath rockets that made strange hissing noises and lit up the night sky over the Syrian border. I wanted to take hold of her hand as we hurried along but didn't dare, didn't want her to realise how scared I was. Then back at the volunteer houses we found a scorpion in the shower room. Rob ushered it out with a broom before we shut all doors tight, checked beds and sleeping bags, clothes and boots as they prefer dark comfy places. And then we turned the lights off and crawled into beds with nerves on edge.

PART III

I'm going to be a doctor"

"Are you?"

"Yes, I'm going to be a doctor"

Isla's got a plastic stethoscope and she's pointing it at me.

"Are you poorly Daddy?"

"I don't feel poorly"

But I know that's no sign.

She swings around.

"Mammy, are you poorly?"

Mammy sighs, just a little bit. Nothing out of the ordinary that would suggest anything other than a game.

"Yes darling, I suppose I am"

So Isla makes her lift her top up and puts a plastic stethoscope on her tummy.

"This will make you better Mammy"

The soldiers came with machine guns out front, not slung over shoulders. We smiled, uncertain. These were our friends, Hanan and Moses. They tried to explain but their English was poor, our Hebrew non-existent. Out the house they ushered us, with serious faces, to the girls' house, gathered us all together in the living room and locked doors, all of us, including them, inside. I looked out the window, saw kibbutzniks hurrying with machine guns to designated places. Moses gestured for me to come away. This was no exercise. The border fence had been breached. "Terrorists" were headed our way. Nobody told ghost stories this time. And we were all very much aware that the volunteer houses were on the far edge of the kibbutz, nearest to the borders. Hanan explained the last time terrorists came across they flew on a hang-glider. He mimicked the actions until someone guessed what he was talking about. They managed to shoot several people dead before getting shot down themselves. The room fell into deathly silence, the rest of the kibbutz too. Not even dogs barked. Then Jane started crying and wrote a letter to her parents stating how much she loved them. I looked at Hanan and Moses, younger than me, and I wondered what went through their heads. I'd already begun to understand why men looked older there. Hagai refused to talk about his three years in the Gaza Strip. Isaac, the eighteen year old son of a kibbutz couple, lay down on the ground the day before and refused to work. It was his last day before joining up. Helen told us earlier that Uzi had shot an Arab in the head after he'd pulled a knife and thrust it towards Hanan's throat. And there we were, on foreign soil, on land taken and held by invading force, out of our depths, in the middle of something you read about in a Sunday morning newspaper with a nice safe cup of tea and slice of toast. I thought I heard the crack of gunfire, but maybe it was my imagination playing games. And then eventually, at half one in the morning, we were allowed out and back in our own houses. At four in the morning we got up for work but were kept in the dining hall and told what had happened. The Golani had shot dead four armed Jordanians in the apple orchards less than half a mile away, the orchards we worked in six mornings a week. We were kept at Afiq while they were searched in the daylight, just to make sure. And then we climbed on the back of the trailer and went to work.

I can be myself at work. I can forget. I can lose myself in the thoughts and worries of creative minds, albeit incarcerated ones. I can answer questions, think up solutions, get frustrated when others can't see their own potential. For two hours in the morning and two in the afternoon, three days per week, I can pretend that everything is normal. I'm not proud of the fact. I wonder if Anna can forget for just one minute. I wonder if it's the last thought on her mind before she eventually falls asleep, her first when she wakes up. I wonder if it's all she thinks about when she's lying there awake most the night. And I understand why sleeping has suddenly become so difficult for her. But for those two hours in the morning and afternoon, my life is as it should be. I can't forget when the classes finish, when I've locked dictionaries and computer leads back in cupboards, when I'm stood around waiting for prisoners to be searched, taken back to cells. I wander over to the barred window, look out into the yard as the movement gets underway; those in green trousers back from the workshops, others from the gym, from education. One with a guitar, three with books and files. A couple move with a swagger and a shout, playing big boys games that got them locked up in the first place. Others slower, hands in pockets, resigned, or maybe relaxed, getting two minutes sun on their faces before being locked up again. Men of all shapes and sizes. Prison officers stood at regular intervals, casting eyes and counting off. It helps you appreciate what you have, working in a prison where many are serving between ten and thirty years. It helps you appreciate your freedom, your loved ones and the time you spend with them. The prisoners disappear into dull brick wings. The officers lock up behind them and my mind returns fully to life on the outside. Some of my colleagues seem scared to ask about Anna, fearful I might tell them it's escalated even further. I understand. Every time I have news it's terrible. Better not to ask. Perhaps they're fearful of their own mortality, caught up in their own worries. We're hardly the only ones with difficulties after all. Or maybe they recognise I don't want to talk about it all the time. But when my colleagues sit around the table talking trivialities or joking with each other, I can't help but think of her, of how I'd cope, of how the children would cope if the worst happened. It's like a trap you can't escape from. You don't want to talk about it but you can't think of anything else most of the time. And almost everything else is irrelevant in comparison anyway.

I come home to find Joe and Isla, their friend Eleanor with her beautiful smile, cut up apples and a house soothing with harmony; Anna, as usual, the graceful conductor. And then I see the package on the table. I take it upstairs, bite cello tape with teeth and out comes two copies of my first novel, sent by the publisher weeks before its actual release. The first one out is Anna's. They're all dedicated to her. If there's a print run of ten thousand then every single one will have a page with the words "For Anna, with love." But this one is her own copy. I write a personal message and take it downstairs with a smile. And it's accepted the way I know it will be; with wonder, love and pride. Then I see Writers News has been delivered too, and when I pick it up I recognise the photograph on the front cover. It's me, with the cover of the book. The front page story and headline belong to me too. "Debut novel provides a life-changing opportunity" it says, explaining how a background of social work and journalism, combined with a publishing deal, has enabled me to work in a prison teaching creative writing. Anna is as pleased as she could be. I pick my book up, stroke its cover front and back, stroke it gently like a small pet, open it and stroke pages, read random words, my acknowledgements and author's note, gaze in wonder at pages like they're works of art. And I take the night for myself. I drink a bottle of wine and claim the night as my own. And Anna is happy for me, is proud of me, is delighted to give me this night.

The 'terrorist' attack was a stark reminder of our environment. On occasions we wondered how nine naive young Brits could sign up for a working holiday and be sent to such a place. But most of us were too involved emotionally and physically to give up so soon. Not Jane and Sarah though; they left for a safer and more sociable kibbutz. We walked them to the bus stop, hugged them goodbye. The German girls left the day before Helen's 24th birthday. Anna and I walked to Bnei Yehuda for cake and candles and Helen cried as we sang to her inside a full dining room. Then Pete left, fed up with the kibbutz lifestyle. Nobody blamed him. He couldn't be bothered with the hassle anymore; the fact volunteers had to wait half an hour after the shop opened so everyone else could clean it out, that we could only buy three packets of cigarettes a month whereas the soldiers could buy twenty-four, that hardly anyone spoke to us. I was sad he was leaving and wanted to see him off but neither he nor Anna woke me, saying I looked happy sleeping. Pete said he wouldn't miss anyone; he never did. I wasn't so sure. I read brilliant letters from friends back home, for the first time thought about missing them, missing family. But we had work to do, adventures to undertake, and I still had Anna, Helen and Rob. We climbed into a banana plantation, stole fruit off the tree but they were foul and unripe. We swam in the Sea of Galilee, made a fire and drank vodka on the beach, slept there as the gentle night breeze rippled our dreams. We found more bunkers and tunnels on the mountainside, more Syrian houses punctured with bullet holes, the remains of what we were told later was a three thousand year old Greek settlement. Anna and I went almost everywhere together but nothing intimate happened. Rob was with us the vast majority of the time, Helen too, when she wasn't spending time with Uzi. I began to think how I should make the first move, began to question and criticise myself for not having done so already. I was afraid of rejection, of humiliation, but was almost sure she felt the same way. I needed alcohol for bravery; that and time for just the two of us.

We're going around the supermarket trying to sly things into the trolley without Isla noticing. It's her third birthday on Tuesday and we're feeling guilty we haven't given it much thought. Anna and I get irritated with each other over who gets what on the shopping list; pathetic and more me as usual. I remind myself I need to be more understanding than I usually am, less prone to sarcasm, to childishness. Then we move towards the till and I look in other peoples trolleys to see what they're buying. Most of them are full of sweet food, convenience food, ready meals and the like. Ours is far healthier. And I think to myself, this isn't fair. This isn't fucking fair.

Seven a.m. and I'm running round the dene and back again. I've had my green tea instead of coffee and I'm pounding the track under trees and squawking crows, Caffrey shuffling along behind me. My knees take the weight and my back feels the strain and I start to wonder if I'm running away or towards something. And then I realise it's both. I'm running away from cancer, from cigarettes and alcohol, from disease and ill health, from myself and my own fears. And I'm running towards good health, towards being in a better place physically and mentally to help Anna and the kids. The other route is at the bottom of a bottle and I know that's not the right path, however tempting it seems at times. Past the stone obelisk that marks the grave of a witch caught in the act of her human rights. But I don't run that far, have to stop before I get back home again, finished by a slight incline that would be too embarrassed to call itself a challenge. And to call it running, well that's a bit of an exaggeration too. But I know when I'm finished and back home that it was the right thing to do, that exercise makes me feel as if I can cope with almost anything. And then I look at Anna and I remind myself it's not me that has cancer, that has to live with the fact cells inside of me are infected and spreading. She sees me looking, smiles warmly, too diplomatic to remark upon my red face and heaving chest. I'm amazed how she continues with such grace and composure. I don't expect it. I wouldn't think any less of her if she broke down. In fact it would make more sense. But she's not the type. Five foot four, slim as a roe deer but filled to the brim with dignity and determination, with thought for others even in such terrible circumstances. Me? I'm just full of admiration, love and respect. I'm not sure I'd be that way.

They cried like babies when you picked them up. They cried like babies when you threw them, when you stood on them. And they often shat on you as well. The soldier I was working with punched Orna's husband in the face, had to be restrained, was thrown out. Orna's husband just carried on where he left off, kicking out, standing on top of them, breaking legs and crushing bodies. I breathed in sawdust and shit, rubbed it out my eyes every two minutes, felt like vomiting, couldn't believe I'd worked a full dayshift then come to this overnight. According to Rob there were fifteen thousand chickens just in my pen, and that didn't seem exaggeration when you were there. He refused, said he was vegetarian. I went along, didn't like to duck a challenge, stood there shin deep in carpet of white feathers and clucking as the gate opened at the far end and a monster of a machine came slowly rolling in. Most of the chickens seemed oblivious at the start; just the odd bit of disturbed fussing down the front. But the machine had arrived under the cover of dark. For all they knew, nothing was different that night. Then its full beam headlights violated every inch of the building and after a second or two of blind paralysis panic started to set in. The mechanical device in front began to rotate round and round, scooping the shaking fowl inside, shoving them into cages at the back. Fussing turned to screams that rose in white topped shuddering waves. My job was simple. I had to ensure all the chickens went inside the machine, get them into the middle of the pen so they could be snatched up and taken to the slaughterhouse. The soldier was on the other side for the first half hour, but when he was escorted out I had to do both sides on my own. By midnight my insides were full of sawdust and shit, my eyes clogged and stinging. Five hours of crying and screaming had drained my emotional energy. Now that most of them were taken, were locked up tight in cages, those left behind hid at the edges of the pen, sheltered their faces from light and noise, clucked with feeble whimper. By one in the morning I'd left encouragement behind and was swinging feet at them, launching them into the air, desperate to get finished and get the fuck out.

It's strong black coffee this morning, to counteract last night's three large glasses of wine, not that they had much of an effect. It's a waste of time drinking alcohol that way, gulping it down before sucks on a cigarette. Large sips of whisky do the job better. I go to the swimming pool with Joe, three other boys and their Dads. Anna takes Isla to her birthday party, a female only princess party the Sunday before her real birth date. Nic and Helen knew nothing was arranged for Isla, that our heads were elsewhere, took it upon themselves to organise everything, arranged for men and boys to go swimming. Told us both when everything was sorted. It was a beautiful idea from beautiful friends. But on the day I want to be with Anna, with my daughter as she opens her presents, blows out candles on the first birthday she really knows about. At home later on, while everyone else is upstairs, I pick up the camera and go through the pictures on it. Isla in her beautiful Chinese dress, all smiles and centre of attention. Ruby dressed as Supergirl, Eleanor as Snow White, Niamh and Eden as fairies. I see cups of juice, princess plates and a homemade hedgehog birthday cake. And I realise Isla didn't miss her Daddy, that she had a wonderful time with all the girls.

The cold wind blowing straight off the grey North Sea fails to dampen the enthusiasm of dozens of young minds and limbs. Inside the new sand dunes playground all is chaos, shouting and laughter, climbing and sliding. I push Isla on the swing, keep an eye on Joe, smile at other parents, pretend I'm happy. On the outside of the new wooden posts, Anna throws a ball for Caffrey and Molly, dark sunglasses hiding her emotions, her movements sluggish and deliberate. I want to reach out, pull her inside and hold her. I want her to be enjoying herself with all the other parents and children, grinning as her children whizz down the new slide, steadying as they climb. I want us to be a normal family again.

I'm making tea. Joe's reading Isla's new library books while his sister colours in Peppa Pig pictures. I feel sick. I want to shout and cry. And I think I can see Anna feeling that way too. You shouldn't feel like this on the weekend you're celebrating your daughter's third birthday. Isla tells me she played pass the parcel, then shows me the box she decorated. Once more, I feel I've totally missed her celebrations, and that I've hardly bought her anything either. Anna says it was lovely but she felt a bit overwhelmed. The rice boils over, shakes the pan lid as white frothy water streams down the outside. Neither of us has got an appetite anyway. And I turn the football off the radio because it's meaningless.

At first there was nothing but barren land and rocky hills. Then we passed through the West Bank and the driver put his foot down. I tried my best to take it all in as they whizzed past; ruined houses half destroyed, walls and fences behind which anyone could be lurking, settlements of tin sheds. Earlier in the year, gunmen had opened fire on a bus here, massacred thirteen people. I wasn't sure if the large assortment of soldiers seated around us made me feel safer or more vulnerable. Then the tin sheds were left behind to be replaced by homemade tents of blankets and sheets, herdsmen coming down hills in Arab costume and headdress, crooks under arm, following goats or cattle. And we came around the corner of a mountain, past a few modern houses and there it was; Jerusalem, just like you've always imagined. Into a taxi after being told it was getting late and dangerous, through dark and narrow streets we went, faster than we might have wished. Past old men sitting out, stray cats dashing, people selling food from cardboard boxes. Until Damascus Gate stood proudly before us, holding up magnificent walls, the entrance to a city since the 4th Millennium before Christ. We climbed old concrete stairs, knocked on the door of the Faisal Hostel. An old Arab guy in white robes and headdress answered, seemed reluctant until we told him we were from Afiq. There was a history of Afiq volunteers staying there, passed down throughout the years. He checked none of us were Jewish as they were banned, introduced himself as Ali, showed us to our rooms. Anna and Helen shared with six other women, Rob and I with a Japanese Buddhist Monk, a member of World Peace Order. We sat on the balcony for a couple of hours, watched Arabs and Orthodox Jews walk past, noticed the presence of Israeli soldiers in dark green uniforms. As sunlight faded we went out for a walk to the mosque at the top of the road but weren't allowed in by security. Then back again and down wide steps to Damascus Gate, built by Suleiman the Magnificent in 1542. Into the narrow confines of the Old City. Five minutes through dark alleys we managed, between the Christian and Muslim Quarters, under ancient tall buildings that leaned across and whispered secrets to each other. The only other people we saw were a group of eight or nine Israeli soldiers looking alert and nervous. And then back to the hostel quick, scared tourists. Rob and I talked to the Buddhist Monk who showed us pictures of a temple in the Himalayas where the opening of Peace Power was held. Anna stayed up speaking to Ali, who worked as a nurse, spent two years in a psychiatric hospital, told her stories of black chickens and brain surgeons.

Joe sings happy birthday to his little sister, kisses and cuddles her. Isla insists he sing happy birthday to Millie her fluffy dog instead. Anna looks on, slightly low cut top showing some cleavage, a section of white dressing.

"You look fantastic," I tell her.

"I want to be smart for Isla's birthday," she says.

I take Joe to school, drop Isla off with Claire the childminder, tell her we may not be back in time to hold a party tea.

Anna puts her best coat on, brings Isla's few but beautifully wrapped presents downstairs, places them carefully by the fireplace. Fifteen minutes later we're on that metro again, Whitley Bay to Haymarket, heads stuck in newspapers. The front page has pictures of Eastenders stars at the funeral of Wendy Richard. We hold hands tight, read more than we usually would. I turn the page, notice horoscopes, need the paper to last as long as possible. Start with my own; Gemini: "if there's help on offer at work, you'd be a fool not to take it. You're trying to struggle valiantly under a heavy load"

Then to Anna's horoscope; Cancer: "very much a home focused day this one, during which you can make lots of progress with DIY projects"

I'm halfway through before I realise Anna isn't Cancer at all. I must have been drawn to that word subconsciously. Anna's Capricorn. But then I realise for what seems like the first time that Joe's star sign is Cancer, and I resent putting those two words together. I finish reading before Anna. One metro station to go and nerves start kicking me in the guts. Anna doesn't realise we've arrived. I tap her on the leg and she looks up, surprised. She's still trying to finish every word.

We pass a young girl with a green face at the hospital gates. She's holding hands with her Mam. Her sad eyes meet ours, then look to the floor. At first I think it's a faded face painting. Then I realise that's actually the colour she is. I wait until we're out of earshot and ask Anna. Jaundice she says. And then we're back in Waiting Room G, but surrounded by different people this time. We sit down, glance around. A middle aged lady's reading The Sun, holding it up in front of her, presumably oblivious to the large print headline she's showing to the rest of the room.

"Jade Goody's Going Blind"

The nerves get stronger. Anna's still reading – anything;

leaflets, magazines, posters on the wall. It doesn't matter if they're interesting or not.

And then another doctor - the fourth one.

Anna strips her top half, lays down on the bed. He pulls the sheet down, feels her breast, the other one. My breathing stops. God knows what's happening inside Anna.

"I'm not worried," he says. "It feels like a cyst"

Anna smiles like she doesn't believe him.

"That's what they said the last time," she says.

After a balcony breakfast of bread, cheese and yoghurt we approached Damascus Gate again, amazed at the changes daylight brought. The steps were full of Arab tradesmen, wares laid out around them. We stepped down past jewellery and pipes, t-shirts and stereos until we were under the gate, imposing towers either side. And then we were inside the   Old City, with barely room to move. People approached from all directions, wanting to take our dollars, our sterling, sell us jewellery, rugs, clothing and pottery. We edged forward, not daring to stop. Some were forceful, tried to lead us into shops with a tug of the arm. Others ran after us, lowering the price as we walked away. I changed twenty dollars on the black market, was taken down a side alley, wondered for a moment if I was doing the right thing. But on we continued, past spices of all colour, past flatbreads and boxes of fruit, fashion and traditional wear, dodging trolleys full of laundry and animal parts, women with baskets on their heads. Lunch was eaten beneath the Mount of Olives. Then over cobbled paving we went, up worn steps, hearing music from both sides of the world; through a narrow tunnel where the lights shone like water on the roof and voices echoed like ghosts from past conflicts. Out into the bright sunshine of a large open square, with the Wailing Wall, built by Herod the Great nineteen years before Christ, still standing strong on the far side. We walked over, more impressed with its size the closer we got, the further we were forced to strain our necks upward. And then down again to orthodox Jews with their backs to us pushing letters to God into its cracks. And our right; an extended family that held hands and span round in a slow Hebrew chanting circle.

The next morning, Anna and Helen went to the bakery to buy cheese but came back with sour cream by mistake. And so it was sour cream and stale bread for breakfast. We found the Dome of the Rock, the oldest surviving Islamic building in the world, built on the site of King Solomon's Temple, who was said to have turned away from God for the lure of incredible wealth, for seven hundred wives and three hundred concubines. Up through the courtyard in expectation we went, past ancient olives trees and elegant carved marble, studying beautiful mosaic tiles, shielding our eyes from the magnificent golden dome. Muhammad ascended to heaven from there, accompanied by the angel Gabriel. Also underneath that rock; the holiest site in Judaism, traditionally regarded by Jews as the holiest spot on Earth. It was closed for prayers. Then Anna and Helen remarked they needed the toilet. An attendant let Anna use the men's but an old Arab guy started shouting when she went in and the next toilet block was locked. So with the girls starting to get a little nervous and desperate, the attendant accepted responsibility and led the way again. Ten minutes later, we were out the Old City, up a street by a long section of grass. Another man shouted across at me, offered ten camels for both Anna and Helen. I agreed, secretly proud at the suggestion I owned them. But the girls wouldn't stop, had other things on their minds. Across the grass we walked, until we saw it at the bottom; a bucket, standing on its own. The attendant looked at the girls, pointed at the bucket, put his lips together and shrugged. Nobody knew what to say for a few seconds. Then the girls refused and after apologies from the man we got back to the hostel just in time. And while the girls stayed for a relieved rest Rob and I went back to the Old City to exchange travellers' cheques and buy some hashish.

We're here again. Outside the Mammography Suite. Only this time Barrack Obama's not on the television; some budget house-buying programme is. I glance at the clock. It's well past midday and Isla's celebrating her third birthday at someone else's house. And we don't know if we'll be able to celebrate with her, because we're already forty minutes late and we're only a third of the way through.

She's only in fifteen minutes this time though, comes back out, says they did the needle test there and then. The sample probably won't get sent to the lab as they're quite sure it's a cyst. Two minutes later, the doctor calls us in, smiles warmly.

"The results were clear. Nothing to worry about"

Anna smiles back.

"Well, not about that one anyway"

We shake hands, say thanks and leave. Good news for a change. Go home to celebrate our daughter's birthday.

Isla's opening presents and Joe's even more excited than she is. Anna's parents, Building Granny and Grandad, are round too. We'd bought Isla some more presents in town and the rest of the day is beautiful. Then Grandad goes for a rest and Granny reads books and helps put kids to bed. Comes downstairs for some serious adult time. I'm on the computer but I hear them talking behind me, in the kitchen. Her Mum talks about losing eyelashes and eyebrows, how make up will help. She's worked in cancer care for almost twenty years, seen hundreds of worst case scenarios. I hear her crying but don't turn around, can almost feel them hugging. Then I drive her Mum back to her flat in North Shields. She gives me two leaflets about what to say to the children, right from the earliest stages all the way through to death. She tells me to hide them from Joe for the time being as there are pictures of children and one of them has the same name as him. And then we hug closely, say we love each other.

We'd exchanged travellers' cheques, were walking back to the Gate of Damascus when they started running towards us; dozens of Arabs frantically trying to get away as fast as they could. Shouts and screams filled what little air there was. Those that walked alongside us also turned and fled. But not Rob and I. We stood there like a pair of fools, frozen to the spot, no experience or precedent for our instincts to fall back on. And we'd arranged to meet this old guy to buy some hashish. I hadn't smoked a joint for nearly two months. So we carried on walking forwards, got within fifteen metres of the scene; four or five Israeli soldiers inside a shop, pushing people about. A large group were gathered outside, shouting and shoving. One of the soldiers must have waved a nervous gun to create some space, sent people fleeing. A young Arab girl made a bolt for it. Out the shop she went but a soldier caught her quick, wrestled her back. A number of Arab guys shouted louder, moved closer. The girl tried to twist free but was held tight. Rob and I looked at each other, decided we'd seen enough, went back the way we came in a fast trot as voices grew harsher behind. Taking the scene as an omen we forgot about meeting the old guy, went back to the safety of the hostel instead. Stories of westerners arranging to buy hashish, then being arrested and imprisoned immediately after, had already unnerved us. And so back on the balcony with the girls we sat, watching the incident spread below. Army jeeps and police pulled up. The soldiers became more aggressive, used elbows and pointed guns when people got too close. Two women were dragged into army jeeps, though we weren't sure why. Then, when everything died down, we went back through the Old City, out the other side, climbed the Mount of Olives and visited the Garden of Gethsemane, where Jesus stayed for twelve hours before he gave himself up for crucifixion. On the way back we went into the Church of the Holy Sepulchre, built on the site of Jesus' crucifixion, including the Tomb of Christ and the prison he was held in. And then Mary's Tomb, filled with enough gold and silver to make her son feel nauseous.

~

Waiting. Waiting. Waiting.

For something terrible to happen.

You know its coming and you know there's nothing you can do but try your best to be positive. Try your best to keep it all together. Though of course it's not me going to experience it. I'm the observer. I'm going to watch it happen to the person I love most in the world. I'm going to be her carer - me, a selfish bugger most of my life. I'm going to be her confidante, her protection. I'm going to tell her I love her when her hair is falling out. And when she loses her eyebrows and eyelashes, when she loses weight and loses more weight, I'm going to tell her I still find her attractive. I'm going to hold her hand and help lead her through.

Because there's nothing else I can do.

A different hospital. Another doctor.

This time an oncologist.

Anna says she feels stronger, more positive now she's had good news about the other breast. The doctor talks about the process, how he picks up the baton after her mastectomy. He explains the side effects of chemotherapy, checks her weight, makes a joke about how she'll be a little bit lighter when she comes in for the chemo. Then gets on the phone, starts arranging. Anna begins to fret, didn't realise things would happen so soon after surgery. When April 9th is mentioned she interrupts.

"Excuse me"

He continues his conversation.

"Excuse me"

He stops, looks across at her.

"I can't start my chemo before April 9th and I definitely can't do anything on that day. It's the launch of Richard's novel"

I start to argue, don't want my launch to get in the way of life or death.

She waives away my protestations, will be there whatever anyone thinks. Everything's put back a week. The doctor smiles, says it will make no difference medically.

I arrive back at ten p.m., have been out since half-six this morning, working at the prison then at Rick Fury's flat practicing our reading and rapping combination for the book launch. Everything went well and I'm full of it. I pour myself a whisky, make a roll up. And I'm outside drinking and smoking, swaggering around the garden like a wannabe rock-star. I walk past the kitchen window and look in. She's at the sink washing plant pots, stacks upon stacks of them, keeping herself busy.

I spend the morning sending e-mails to local press while Anna takes Isla to playgroup. I get an answer within two hours, an upcoming interview and feature. Then Anna comes back and is subdued the rest of the day. When the kids are in bed I take loads of baby gear round to her brother.

She spent hours in the loft last night, sorting through it. Then I come back and we sit on the couch together, hold hands and talk about the next few days. The weekend is arranged; who to see and what to do. It's a weekend to look forward to. Anna says she's not down, just tired, though she is worried her cancer will spoil the birth of Richard and Louise's first child. But when I look into her eyes I'm not sure I believe her. She's having her breast cut off on Thursday. She doesn't want to put a downer on all my good news, start moving down the wrong direction in case it's a one way street. She goes to bed but knows it will take hours before she falls asleep. I pour myself another whisky and eat some more of her chocolate.

Ali hugged us goodbye. We boarded the bus, squeezed into seats and sat back for the ride, trusting Rob's advice that En Gedi really was a popular tourist resort. Back through the West Bank we sped, finding out later the same number bus was machine gunned the day before. Five killed and plenty more injured. Over some mountains, down to the shore of the Dead Sea we went, as darkness finally settled on the lowest point on earth. The driver dropped us off, disappeared into the dust. We put our bags down and looked around; one youth hostel and nothing else. So we walked up to the youth hostel and knocked. A man answered, said it was thirty-six shekels each, told us not to sleep outside because leopards had killed three dogs the previous night. We wondered if he was trying to scare us out of our money but it didn't matter; we didn't have enough anyway. And leopards didn't exist in Israel, surely. Then a girl came by and told us not to sleep on the beach because Jordanian terrorists sailed over under cover of the night. We had a beer each and some biscuits, didn't have enough for a whole meal, went down to the shore in the pitch black, stripped to our underwear and waded in. Our legs floated up when the water reached our waists. We pretended to ride bikes, sat up in armchairs, laughed then laughed some more, giddy with the experience. We reached down and grabbed handfuls of mud, wiped it onto our skin like Cleopatra over two thousand years before. And then, accustomed to salt that burned scratches, we floated in silence, looked up at thousands of stars, the Jordanian mountains on the other side. And we wondered if we fell asleep whether or not we would wake up on the shores of another country.

Greasy and sticky was how we came out though, covered in a slimy film of salt. We decided to wash at the youth hostel but they wouldn't let us in. So we found a tap outside and washed our hands and faces in cold water, leaving hair matted from salt and starting to dread. And then, with cold and tiredness starting to creep in, myself and Anna went looking for firewood that wasn't encrusted with salt and so would burn. After an hour's scavenging over barren land we held a paltry amount in our arms and had been stopped twice by soldiers in jeeps with headlights that blinded us. Our fire was appalling. It fizzled to a pathetic halt minutes after Rob made everyone paranoid by saying he'd spotted a scorpion. We laid our two sleeping bags on the sand, cuddled up to each other for body warmth. The desert night penetrated our bones and Helen sang songs until we eventually drifted asleep.

Isla climbs sleepily into our bed, into the middle as always. We stroke her lovingly, the most beautiful girl in the world. Normally I'd be the one to rub her tummy, touch her face, stroke her hair. But I back off this time, allow Anna instead. She needs it more than I do. Isla picks hands up from underneath the duvet, asks who they belong to. Finds she's got one of each. Let's go of mine, turns her back on me.

"I want to hold two of Mammy's hands," she says.

Joe is Iron Man and I'm Hawk Eye.

"Come on, let's go," he says in a perfect American accent.

Isla decides her and Mammy are playing a different game. She's Fifi Flowertot while Mammy is Bumble the Bee. We walk together, two games existing simultaneously. Occasionally the bee buzzes off. Not for long, just ten seconds or so, lost in her own world until Fifi's insistence brings her back again. I watch over my shoulder as she's dragged back into the present by a three year old. She never used to be like that. Then we're on the beach and the bee has become Anna again. She builds a boat out of sand, makes a maze out of washed up sticks. Joe and I wander off, dodge acid seawater, investigate strange markings. I collect sea coal and shells for the path around the vegetable beds, watch oyster catchers run away from us, all beautiful bodies and comedy legs. Then we're back with the girls and Joe climbs into the boat with Isla, joins in their game. Anna adds stick levers and shell buttons, turns an old washed up barbecue into a Sat Nav system. I throw a stick for Caffrey, engage in a growling tug of war, look back at Anna and the children, then turn to the sea. The tide is out as far as it can go; ripples flat and gentle. The early spring sun warms my face, brushed by a cool breeze. I walk over, grab Anna around the waist, kiss her back and neck. It's a perfect moment. It's what Sundays were made for.

Joe and Isla are at school and nursery. Two newspapers are interviewing me later and a photographer's coming round as well. I've dreamed about days like this for years. But tomorrow is the day of Anna's mastectomy and we're arguing. She's cleaning downstairs while I'm trying to do some last minute reading and thinking so I don't make a fool of myself. Anna warns about my pile of clothes in the bedroom again. Says I need to prepare what meals I'll be cooking for the children. I fret and shout, can't deal with domesticity and interviews at the same time, escape upstairs, sort my hair out, replace an old jumper with a shirt. Anna finishes cleaning the floor, is putting things back when the photographer arrives. He takes a few pictures by the laptop, the fireplace. I'm nervous at first, self-conscious. But then we go out and he takes dozens of pictures in a back alley, me leaning on a lamppost looking all serious. Within minutes I'm confident, happy. This is what I want. I could pose all day, forget everything else. But I have to go back home and deal with reality.

Anna collects Joe from school. I take Caffrey along the cliffs, down the winding path onto rocks. There's not a cloud to be seen, just beautiful blue sky highlighting sea that laps the pebble shore. People yearn for holidays abroad, rave about the Highlands, The Lake District. But here I am between Newcastle and Blyth, often referred to as some kind of industrial heartland. And it's beautiful. At times as beautiful as anywhere could be. And somehow, now one of my loved ones is close to death, my senses and appreciation of nature seem even more heightened. And if I could do this, walk here with Anna until old age, over beach and dune, dene and cliff, round the harbour and across to St Mary's Island where it's said mermaids were once frequent visitors. If I could do all this I would give everything else up, all my dreams and frustrations. To be stripped of everything that's superfluous, all those glittering accessories that mean nothing in the wider scheme of things, all that's ego enhancing and judged by monetary value. To be left with all that's most necessary – love and life, health and family. I return by the back of Joe's school, look out over the playing field, see my boy with his friends on the wooden Viking ship. Anna, further back, with a couple of mams, as if everything was normal. As if nothing had happened.

Like nothing will happen.

The sun rose imperiously over the mountains of Jordan, bringing dark red sheets that reflected off the Dead Sea. We missed the five-thirty a.m. bus because we were too cold to move, ran after the six a.m. bus, our bodies cracking in salt. It disappeared around the corner of a mountain before we could reach it. The next bus didn't arrive for over two hours so we unpacked our sleeping bags and waited at the bus stop, next to a sign that read "Beware of leopards. Hitchhike in groups of four or more." After changing money in Jerusalem, Helen and Rob caught the bus to Tiberius but Anna and I had other ideas. We wanted to explore together before she went back to England. Our plan was to move to another kibbutz with or without others, not realising, or perhaps not yet fully accepting, we could have the most wonderful time at Afiq if we admitted our growing interest and explored each other instead. And so Anna and I got off the bus at Tel Aviv with no address for the kibbutz office, no map, one bar of chocolate and a bag of banana chips. Tourist information didn't know where the kibbutz office was. We found the post office and though the staff didn't speak English they wrote 'Sutin 10' on a piece of paper. So we started walking and asking directions and within twenty minutes got three different finger points, were told it was three kilometres away, five kilometres away and twelve kilometres away. Eventually we found the street after an hour and a half walking but it was a block of residential flats. We shrugged and smiled, frustrated and shattered but happy to have each other for company. Who knows; perhaps, in that mutual silence, we made an unconscious pact to stop exploring outwards and look a little closer to home.

We missed the eleven a.m. bus because we didn't want to put out newly bought cigarettes. Then, boarding the eleven-thirty I realised I'd lost or had stolen fifty shekels and my camera. That meant we didn't have enough money to get back to Tiberius, never mind the kibbutz. So we bussed it to Afula which was all we could afford. And then, nervous in an unfamiliar Arab town, with most of our experiences being around Jewish people, we had no choice but to hitchhike. The minibus seemed like any other vehicle to us. We climbed in alongside others, didn't think twice. Five kilometres later, the driver demanded money. He wanted forty shekels but we only had two between us. He shouted at us, stabbed his finger to emphasise his disgust. Stopped and threw us out. At one point that night we thought we'd have to sleep the night rough. But eventually we got back to Afiq with six different lifts; an orthodox Jew with his young baby, a soldier who spoke no English but managed to cadge two cigarettes, a labourer who took us to Tiberius, a huge lorry that took us to Zemah and an Arabic guy who took us to Bnei Yehuda. We walked the last few kilometres and got back at ten p.m., six hours after setting off. Exhausted, we told our story with relieved grins, soaked up laughter from other volunteers. Checked the work list and realised we had to be up at four-thirty a.m. the next day. Then we collapsed into beds, not realising our luck with hitchhiking was about to run out in the most terrifying of circumstances.

Isla points out the car window.

"Daddy, can you buy me one of those?"

I glance out. It's an old man on a mobility machine.

"No darling. They're for people whose legs don't work properly"

She slumps back in her car seat and groans.

"Who's putting me to bed tonight?"

"I am"

"Aaaawww; not Mammy?"

"No darling, sorry. And guess what? Guess who's putting you to bed tomorrow night?"

"Who?"

"Building Granny and Aunty Louise"

"Why?"

"Because Mammy's going to hospital and Daddy will be visiting her. So you'll get Building Granny and Aunty Louise to read your stories. That's good isn't it?"

"Why's Mammy going to hospital again?"

"Because she's having another lump taken out darling. Except this one's a bit bigger. But it will stop her getting poorly so that's good"

I wonder what we'll say when Mammy's hair starts falling out. When the chemo starts to steal all her energy.

Isla thinks for a moment. I can see her in the rear view mirror, eyes moving around her head, trying to make sense of things.

"Big Bobby needs a wee"

"What?"

She's cuddling him; a large white teddy bear.

"You have to stop the car. Big Bobby needs a wee"

"Ah, we'll be back in five minutes. I'm sure he can wait"

"He can't wait"

"I'm sure he...."

"You have to stop the car NOW Daddy"

So I do as I'm told. And she takes Big Bobby for a wee at the side of the road.

Helen pops round to make sure she knows what she's doing when Anna's in hospital, and when exactly she's having Joe and Isla. She tells me I can take washing round to hers whenever I want. Notices Anna's look, points at her.

"Don't listen to her. It's going to be a busy time for you. Bring washing round anytime. It's no bother"

Then the kids are in bed and I'm emptying the dishwasher and I'm emotionally and physically drained all of a sudden. The excitement of interviews and photographs has worn off and the reality of tomorrow is upon me. But my train of thought is disturbed by banging upstairs. I march up. Joe says he's not banging. Or walking about. Or playing. He's counting up to four hundred and he was up to three hundred and thirty six and I've just interrupted him so he's going to have to start all over again. I come down and see Anna has her bags ready, has written my lists, has already had a shower, washed hair and painted toe-nails. She asks if I'm alright. I smile and nod my head.

"Don't worry," she says. "It's not a sad day tomorrow, it's a good one. It needs to come off"

I nod. I don't feel sorry for myself. I feel sorry for her. I can't play famous writers anymore but the last few weeks have reminded me there are things in life more important. The time has almost come. We go to bed and cuddle into each other.

Eagles circled where men feared to tread, between high barbed wire fences that separated countries at states of war and suspicion. We watched them, six or seven, away from land and its complications, riding thermals of freedom, brushing wings wider than the height of men through cotton clouds. I wondered if their eyes, eight times more powerful than our own, were fixed on us, a perfect predator that can take down wolves and cattle sizing up the destroyer of its planet. We smoked cigarettes, ate green skinned oranges, listened to the start of the peace conference with the Golani, though most of it was unintelligible to those that didn't understand Hebrew. The four a.m. start had taken a while to recover from but the dawning of our environment brought us to our senses. The avocado orchards were twenty minutes' drive from the kibbutz, as near to the borders as humanly possible. One hill Jordan. One hill Syria. Our hill Israeli occupied. We could have thrown a stone at the border fence from where we were but it wouldn't have been recommended. The occasional tank rolled by, slow moving jeeps fronted and backed by walking soldiers, machine guns at the ready. After listening to the radio and talking loudly to themselves for ten minutes, the soldiers explained parts of the peace process, said there was no chance Israel would give back the Golan Heights to be bombarded by Syria again. They told us six Israeli Defence Force were killed yesterday, three of them Golani who'd been stationed on Afiq the previous year and were personal friends of many that lived there. They pointed out glinting of sunlight on enemy hills, said it was the reflection of binoculars trained upon us.

The alarm goes off at five forty-five a.m. I make Anna a cup of tea as she can't drink anything after half six. But she's not allowed milk so it's peppermint tea. Isla climbs in the middle, cuddles us both, groans when reminded about Mammy going into hospital. I read her Apple Tree Farm, take Caffrey out while Anna encourages children and her mind adjusts to the coming day. Round the harbour I pass another man I see quite often, walking his dog. We usually chat about weather, dogs, his horses, nothing more than that, if we actually stop at all. But once you've started a pattern it seems rude to carry on straight past, and the dogs always run up to each other like long lost friends. So I stop. But we talked about weather yesterday and it's exactly the same this morning. Clear blue sky, calm sea, tide in. And so I tell him. There's a second or two of silence and it just comes out. I say I'm glad it's a fine day because I'll be walking round Newcastle for hours. He looks at me and wonders. I tell him Anna's going for a mastectomy today. And he looks gutted. I don't know if he's ever spoken to Anna, if he even knows what she looks like. But he looks absolutely crestfallen. And I realise I've done the wrong thing. I had no need to tell him, no need to ruin his day, perhaps evoke memories of someone he knows, someone he once knew. So I tell him about the interviews and the photographer and we pursue that for a few minutes instead before going our own ways. Then I look at my watch and realise the taxi's coming in five minutes and I'm still by the harbour. I put Caffrey on the lead and jog. The taxi's outside when I get home, Anna at the door looking down the street. She comes back inside with me, does her hair quickly, cuddles the children, then me. Rushes out like she's going on holiday and doesn't want to miss the plane. I stand at the front door and watch her climb in. She looks back and smiles before shutting the door but I'm sure I can detect a tear seeping out. The driver speeds off before she even has a chance to do her seat belt. I walk back inside, look out the living room window at the space where the car was, where she was. And then a text comes through:

Love you x Love Joe x Love Isla x Love Caffrey x

I reply, tell her we all love her loads too, then go upstairs to our bedroom, straighten the duvet, sit Anna's teddy I bought for her last birthday carefully on her pillow and help Isla get dressed.

Two hours later I take Joe to school, hand a subdued Isla over to Claire, receive words of encouragement from friends and parents, a sympathetic glance from Joe's teacher. Then I walk home, tidy up the children's toys, send another text to Anna even though I know she can't have her mobile turned on in hospital. There's no radio on for distraction today. That would be wrong. I go upstairs in silence, make the children's beds, put their pyjamas on radiators for later, put my pile of clothes away and leave the house.

That metro again...

I sit opposite a young couple with a toddler in between them, all three of them hoodied up. The Daddy helps his son race cars off the seat and into the buggy while talking to the Mam about a school reunion. Then the boy stops racing, cuddles into his Daddy with closed eyes, gets kissed on face and head. Ten seconds later he opens his eyes. He didn't need sleep, just confirmation of love. Then he goes to high five his Daddy but misses and slaps the window. His Mam watches, eyes sparkling with love. I feel happy for them. It makes me want to cry. They get off at Ilford

Road and an old man with a walking stick takes their place. Then it's back to hospital corridors again, and all those scary name plates: Teenage Cancer Trust Unit, Neurophysiology, Haemophilia Centre, Coronary Care Unit, Programmed Investigations Unit, Department of Anaesthesia, Renal Unit. All the way to Ward 31. Except I've got it wrong. It's Ward 39 I should be at. Ward 31 is where she'll go after surgery. So it's back down more corridors until I find her. She's sat in a chair with one of those NHS gowns on, same Paris Hilton stockings as before, hasn't eaten for twenty hours, nothing to drink for seven.

I walk over, kneel down next to her, take hold of her hand and search her eyes.

"How are you?"

She smiles.

"Bored"

"Mmmm, I bet you are"

"Bored and very hungry"

I smile, secretly pleased she doesn't want to talk about surgery. Isn't freaking out, getting all emotional.

"It will all be finished in a few hours darling"

"No it won't be"

"Well no....not all of it, but this stage will be"

She looks to the wall.

"I'm not hungry. I'm starving"

And for some reason this makes me burst out laughing.

"A Thai curry," she says, moving tongue over lips. "I can taste one"

"Yeah, well you can't have one I'm afraid"

"Christmas dinner. With all the trimmings. Steak and chips. With mushrooms and onion rings"

"We'll have something lovely to eat when you get out darling. Whatever you want"

"A cup of tea. Even a cup of tea would do"

But then the nurse comes to interrupt her dreams and take her away for the anaesthetic. An hour later, I'm sat in the same coffee shop as before, a chocolate chip muffin instead of almond. The sun's pouring through the window and Anna's under the knife again. Except this time the knife is going deeper and further. And the turgid pop singer is female.

I laid awake in my sleeping bag, wishing I had Anna's warm body next to mine, as the thunder growled and lightning burst through the window. Still, we would have the coming day off surely. It would be dangerous to climb trees in pouring rain, and lightning killed two people the last time it struck the Golan. At five in the morning we were given waterproofs and told to get on with it. Each time we picked an avocado it brought a freezing cold shower down our necks and backs. On the night Rob and I decided to spend some time together. We walked towards the Syrian border but hardly spoke a word to each other, awkward silence exaggerated by ponderous footsteps in the dark, Rob's torchlight struggling to lead the way. Someone was coming between us and we didn't feel comfortable enough to bring her into conversation. Rob was becoming a lemon and we both knew it. Helen had gone to visit Uzi's mother near Haifa. The fantastic four were splitting apart through love and he was the only one without any. Our bonding mission failed. We decided to head back but were stopped by a screeching noise in the near darkness that sounded neither animal nor machine. Eventually Rob managed to highlight it; a cat with both back legs broken. He tried to move it from the middle of the road but it spat and scowled, scraped legs two yards further up, the sound of bone on concrete raking through our spines. And so we left it on the road to get ran over instead. Two minutes later a car passed. I listened for a crunch but didn't hear one. Thirty seconds later the howling started. We froze, hypnotised like rabbits caught in headlights. It sounded like five or six of them; getting closer. I wondered if they had the taste of blood and flesh on their lips from mangled cat and hurried on faster.

They have a particular smell, hospitals, don't they? Like swimming pools. Only...well, more clinical and deadly I suppose. I pass Anna's surgeon on the way up the stairs, dressed in green robes, white mask around his neck. Just finished cutting someone open and off for a coffee break. He nods his head, says hello, doesn't offer any words of encouragement. I carry onto ward 31, wash my hands and take a seat outside to wait for visiting time.

She's lying on the bed, a drip taking blood and fluid from her wound into a bottle, two plugs sticking out her hands.

Morphine eyes. I tell her she looks fine.

She smiles weakly.

"You do, honest"

"It's the drugs. You get loads this time because it's far more painful"

We chat, say we love each other. I tell her I'm going to have fish to eat on our wedding night and we both remember the fish restaurant we found in Turkey. How we've never eaten better before or after. We decide we won't buy wedding rings beforehand, but take a risk and buy them there. Wander around some old towns and markets. Then I tell her about a campervan I saw in Whitley Bay, how we'll travel the whole coast of Britain. Anna says after the chemo, when she's better, she'd be happy just to walk around Budle Bay, remember the times we came up from inner city London and holidayed in Northumberland. I agree, as long as we can go up Roseberry Topping in the Cleveland hills too, a place that brings back memories of my Gran and Grandad. And then it's time. In fact it's ten minutes over. She gets extra morphine syringed into her bloodstream. We kiss goodnight and say goodbye. And she's closed her eyes before I've turned to leave.

We were moved out the avocado orchards for a while. I worked in the gardens, bemusing Marla who couldn't understand why I didn't want shelter from pouring rain. But I was happy, driving tractor with trailer, trimming bushes and hedges, pruning roses. Climbing onto roofs to pull tangled ivy. Kibbutz dogs followed wherever I went. Six or seven young pups rolling over and play fighting, Eres the leader of their already notorious gang. They stole everything they could; shoes, tools, whatever they could get their paws on, their teeth into. They ran after people and snapped at their heels, hid and jumped out at them, were thrown out the dining hall and laundry on a daily basis. Many kibbutzniks hated them but we loved them and they reciprocated, often waiting for us to finish work and then running round in barking circles at the sight of us. And as for that rain; well it just made me feel more alive. Anna wasn't so lucky. She was put in the laundry, washing and folding clothes for seven hours each day before coming back fed up. But I had plans that would be sure to lighten her mood. I went to Piq one night as soon as I'd finished working in the gardens. I went to wait for her, had decided this should be the place, that the time must be as soon as possible. I found a kingfisher feather inside a bombed house, kept it in my pocket for her. Walked a little way down the valley, smoked a cigarette underneath pomegranate trees surrounded by cattle with birds on their heads. Watched deer running up slopes. Looking back up at the bombed houses as the sun started to fall below the Galilee I waited for her silhouette, was sure she'd come, would know where I was, would need me in her frustration. My mind played possibilities. I would wave at her to climb down. Even better; I'd climb up to where she was and we'd lie on the roof and kiss under a sky that turned blood orange. It was the perfect moment, the perfect place, not fumbling drunk on stolen wine. But she never turned up, even though she must have known where I was, that I was alone. So I climbed back up the valley in deepening darkness, nervous about getting the right foothold, about the strange animal noises that emerged from all around me. And I walked back to the kibbutz alone.

I'm awake before the children, have been awake most of the night. It's usually Anna who can't sleep, who tosses and turns. But it's only the third night Anna has been away from the house since Joe was born nearly six years ago. She's used to being on her own, had to get used to it. I worked overnight every week at the homeless hostel, had training in Liverpool, made the odd festival. Took homeless teenagers sailing round the Channel Islands and on the North Sea. But last night I slept at home and had to leave the light on. I slept on Anna's side of the bed and cuddled her teddy.

Isla climbs in with that beautiful smile, that enthusiasm for the start of a new day. She comes right over and cuddles up, then looks to a space where her Mammy should be and frowns. We make the drinks as usual, but this time there's no Earl Grey to go with black coffee and warm milk. I wonder if Anna had any sleep. Perhaps she's having a dream right now where everything is normal and life is taken for granted like it used to be? Isla chooses her book: Whoever Heard of a Tiger in a Pink Hat? And then I let her choose clothes as well. Do purple and blue match? I'm not sure. The hairclips certainly don't, and Isla has to guide me putting them in.

I put my hands on her shoulders.

"Stand still. Face me"

I smile. She looks like her Daddy got her ready.

I swing my boy through the corridors of the RVI, then decide it's probably not appropriate when he nearly crashes waist height into a nurse coming around the corner. On we go, me gripping his hand tight enough to stop him running. He's excited about seeing his Mammy. Anna looks fantastic. She shouldn't perhaps, but she does. Sat up in cool clothes, a little bit of make-up, toe-nails painted, hair done. Like she's on holiday or something. Now the plugs have been taken from her hands it's easy to miss the tube coming from her wound, falling by her side. Draining blood to a bottle on the floor, discreetly placed inside a small gift bag by the nurses. After cuddles and kisses and Joe giving Anna his mother's day card early because he insists, I extend a finger and pull forward the neckline of the top she bought last week. She's got a large dressing where a breast used to be, a tube coming out, but the skin around the dressing looks normal. We gently cuddle and kiss. I stroke her leg and tell her she looks sexy and it's true, she does. Joe does the dot-to-dot book his Mammy gives him, is impressed with a telly that moves about in mid-air. I want to lie down with her, snuggle in carefully, go to sleep holding her, but I'm not allowed on the bed.

A beautiful spring day. Anna would be desperate to get outside, walk the dog and children, do some gardening. We go to Collywell Bay, the three of us, collect shells and stones for her, do rock climbing riskier than she would allow. Coming back home I realise I forgot to get them to brush their teeth. And we giggle at the thought of their Mammy's disapproval. After dinner, Joe goes to a party at St

Mary's lighthouse and Isla and I drive to the metro station. We get to the hospital ten minutes early so do 'massive jumps' off the statue of Queen Victoria. Then in we go and Isla gives her Mammy homemade cards from Arthur and Eleanor before eating all her grapes. She's never looked more beautiful in my eyes, Anna. Her hair's immaculate. I wish I'd appreciated it more. I wish I could stay too but Isla's been promised fish and chips and it's the end of visiting time. Anna walks out with us to get some fresh air and say goodbye. Isla lies on the pavement and won't get up, refuses bribes of cuddles and kisses from her Mammy, won't come with her Daddy. Says she wants to go back to hospital. I pick her up and walk off with her, legs kicking bruises into me. At the end of the street she shouts "Bye Mammy" at the top of her voice. Then, we're on the metro and she sits on my knee, cuddles in and sucks her thumb. Makes baby noises all the way home.

PART IV

Friday nights were always the most likely. Fuelled by wine already drunk, by excuses of hard work with ridiculous pay and lesser treatment, by intentions not yet revealed, we tip-toed through the dining hall, into the kitchens. Came back out with eleven bottles of wine between four of us. Anna and I stuck to each other all night, so when the decision came to 'borrow' some bikes it was a foregone conclusion that she and I would share. Around the houses we walked until we saw some outside the bomb shelter disco. Rob and Sharon chose one each, took off faster and lighter. Anna sat on the seat, put her hands on my hips. And off we went too, careering around deserted paths, the wind in our hair, funnelling down throats to mix with wine as we tipped our heads back to laugh. Towards the far end of the kibbutz we went, where houses were fewer, where the path stretched longest, from behind the volunteer houses all the way past kibbutznik houses and onto the Bronx where the soldiers lived. We lined up alongside each other, beamed like dragsters, revved plastic handlebars. Then, with feet pressing down on pedals, with gritted teeth and hardened calves lined with stolen red wine veins, we raced each other down the path, past scorpions and snakes hiding under dusty rocks, Rob and Sharon speeding ahead but myself and Anna just behind, her hands holding my waist tight as a lover's clench. Rob and Sharon took a sharp left, looked back and screamed in delight.

"Come on," shrieked Sharon.

But I kept going forwards, along the side of kibbutznik houses, still straight, still picking up speed. I was Evil Knievel. I was Steve McQueen. I was Clyde with Bonnie hanging on for dear life at the back, her fingers gripping tighter, nails digging into skin. The path was coming to an end but my speed still increased.

"Turn left," Anna shouted. "Turn left"

I carried on forwards, the garden and house approaching fast.

"Turn left…"

We hit the hedge full on. The bike stopped but we didn't. Over the handlebars we went, over the hedge too. Then we hit the grass on the other side, alcohol numbed muscles ensuring nothing broken. And as we rubbed our heads and came up onto knees our eyes met and we knew instantly what was going to happen. We embraced and kissed, fell back down onto earth, rolled over on top of each other.

"Let's go back to the house," smiled Anna, aware we were in someone's front garden.

We pulled the bike out the hedge and cycled back towards the volunteer houses, a little slower but urgent with lust. We dumped it before we got there and went straight to Anna's room. Where we undressed and consumed each other.

You think you're on top of things and then you realise the kids are going to bed in ten minutes and their rooms are still trashed. I phone Anna and she sounds flat. And I don't know what to say because I'm flat too. The kitchen and dining table are trashed, the living room too. I've been out nearly all day, not had time to do anything. I put the kids to bed one at a time, read their books, encourage them to wash faces, brush teeth. But I'm tired and grumpy and shout at them. I answer texts, bring the washing in from outside, hang it up. Empty the dishwasher, fill it again, feed the dog and clear up. I can't be bothered to do any of it. Then I remember all those times I sat on the computer and let someone else do it all, even though she was already shattered and hadn't stopped all day.

Half an hour later, Joe shouts me up. Neither he nor Isla have been able to sleep.

"Can I ask you something Daddy?"

"Of course"

"Does Santa live forever?"

I don't know how to answer him. I was going to say no one lives forever but was scared he might ask about his Mammy being in hospital. Anna would know the right thing to say. I tell Joe I don't know and he looks disappointed with me.

We put our heads under the duvet, hide from scary monsters, look at each other with sparkling eyes.

Then Isla looks quizzical.

"What's that on the end of your nose Daddy?"

"I don't know"

"What is it?"

I scratch my nose.

"I can't feel anything"

"I think its fish and chips," she says.

I tickle her. She laughs a few seconds, then suddenly stops.

"Am I seeing Mammy today?"

I stroke hair from out of her face

"I hope so"

"In the hospital?"

"No darling. You're going to Richard and Louise's with Joe. And I'm going to the hospital to see if the doctor will let Mammy come home"

"Will he?"

"I don't know sweetheart. I hope so. It's Mother's Day today so maybe he will"

"What?"

"It's Mother's Day darling. A day when people remember how lovely their Mammy's have been to them"

I picture Anna sat up in her hospital bed. She'll be

desperate to come home. I know she will. But they won't let her leave with a drip in. Not with little children. It won't make any difference to the doctor that it's Mother's Day.

We took our delicate stomachs for a walk down the valley, held hands as we ambled along past tortoise, climbed up past deer and coyote. Soon, we would make love in this valley, by the trickling stream and the kingfisher, hidden by prickly pear cacti we would peel and eat, pricking our fingers and licking off blood. But for now, lost in each other's worlds, we wandered hand in hand until it became dark. And then, forgetting where paths were, we took a different route and walked back up to the top of the valley through the middle of a minefield.

Work alternated between gardens and avocado orchards, or at least it did for me. I cut down hedges and trees, cleared rubbish from the perimeter fence so guards could see without obstruction. Uncovered scorpions and diamond backed snakes, watched eagles fly down from Jordan. Anna folded clothes in the laundry. Sunsets clouded over and Terry Waite was released. We went to the Syrian House and talked for hours but our hands stayed by our sides. The next day Anna came back from the laundry and threw the clothes from her cupboard onto the floor, smashed a bottle and fell onto the bed in tears. It was her period making her emotional she said. That and the thought of spending her last month working inside a laundry. It was nothing to do with me. I felt useless, let Helen deal with it, spent an hour trying to read a book then went to see Marla to ask her to move Anna out the laundry. Back at the girls house I told Anna she was in the dining room the next day. It wasn't perfect but it was a start. We cuddled and kissed but Rob came back with a scratched eye and Anna went to hospital with him. Helen and I watched them go for a lift then talked for three hours, her in charge of topics. She started on travelling. I thought she was going to ask if she could come along with me when Anna went to Newcastle. But she didn't. And then she changed the topic to soul mates, asked what I thought of them.

"I don't know," I said. "I haven't really thought about it before"

She smiled.

"I think there's somebody out there," she said. "Somebody for everyone. Someone who's the perfect match. You just have to try and find each other"

I told her about my Daddy dying when I was two, my Mam marrying again when I was six. Helen talked of the time her Dad came to college to tell her he'd been having an affair and was moving out the family home. She brushed away tears with her sleeve, then told me she had an infected womb, might have to go back to England for an operation.

I listened for a few moments, didn't know what to say. When she stalled for good I changed the topic.

"How's things with Uzi?"

She looked like she was going to cry again.

"Intense," she said, then waited a few seconds to collect herself.

"He's finished his army service in a month's time. He should be happy. He should be looking forward to the rest of his life"

"I take it he isn't then?"

"No. He doesn't have a clue what to do with himself. He's relied on his mates for years and now he's going to be on his own and he's scared"

I smiled sympathetically, began to readjust my stereotypes. Uzi was a thick set, tough looking bear of a lad.

"And he's haunted by nightmares," said Helen. "Of the things he's seen and the things he's done"

"Like shooting that Arab who pulled a knife on Hanan?"

She shook her head.

"It didn't happen that way. Nobody pulled a knife on Hanan. He shot the Arab by mistake. They were throwing bottles at his jeep. In situations like that, when they're not in immediate grave danger, they're supposed to use plastic bullets. But he picked up real ones and shot one of them in the stomach"

"Did he kill him?"

"No, thankfully. But he was charged by the army and got a month in prison. And the prison was a one man tent inside an iron cage, set on its own. He had to stay in there for the whole month. Eat, sleep, piss and shit in there. With nothing to do, no books or paper. Nothing at all. He said the only way to keep sane was to talk to himself about anything, about everything. And to do push ups to keep himself in shape. Then when he came out he had to spend two weeks walking round a thick muddy field pulling a heavy rake on his shoulders and he still wasn't allowed to speak to anyone"

She used my silence to change the topic, revert back to the first one, took me off guard.

"You and Anna are soul mates," she said. "You're meant to be with each other. It's obvious to everyone"

"Is it?"

She laughed. "Yeah, course it is"

It made me feel nervous, her saying that. A vulnerable and beautiful girl who'd paired up with an emotionally damaged solider two thousand miles from home.

She carried on though, still hadn't made her main point.

"If you asked her to go travelling with you, she'd do it at the drop of a hat"

I thought about it a few seconds.

"How can I?"

"What do you mean, how can you?"

"She's got her career all planned out. Everything's arranged. I'm going to miss her loads and loads but I don't want to screw her life up, make her miss her nursing"

She looked to the ground. I was young and I'd never fallen in love before. And I didn't realise just how much I would miss her.

I drop Joe and Isla off at Richard and Louise's, get the metro, ring from Marks and Spencers. Anna doesn't want anything. She's not hungry, just feels sick. Get here as soon as possible she says. Her drip's out. The doctor says she can come home. I make my way to the hospital as fast as I can, pass a pretty nurse eating an apple in the corridor, think of that rhyme, wonder if it keeps the doctor away from her. My eyes start to well as I get closer to Ward 31. She's on the edge of her bed, bags packed, looks pale. Ten minutes later she's got six boxes of medication, lots of well wishes from nurses and we're off. We pick Joe and Isla up from Richard and Louise's, sneak some dinner that wasn't meant for us. The doctor wanted her to stay in a day extra but agreed to her coming home after she did a bit of begging. She was missing her children she said, couldn't sleep. Was so bored.

But when we pull onto our drive she looks like she's going to burst out crying. And this is one of those moments. Even the kids are completely silent.

"At least I've made it back today," she says quietly.

I smile.

"Yeah. Good day too. What with it being Mother's Day and all that"

But she doesn't respond the way I expect her to. Just sits there lost in thought. Then looks at me, seems surprised by my expression.

"What?" I ask her.

"Didn't you hear?"

"Hear what?"

"Jade Goody's dead. I know people slag her off and say she's irritating but that's not the point is it? Her children will never see her again. She died this morning"

Isla and Joe are arguing because they both want their Mammy to read them their bedtime stories. Ordinarily we alternate but tonight I'm happy for the rejection. I stand at the door, lean on the frame and watch her read to them together. Isla sits on her right knee, Joe next to her on the floor. It will be a while before anyone can sit on her left knee, cuddle in that side. Within half an hour they're fast asleep. And an hour later Anna and I are pulling back the covers. A lucky family. A full house again.

Anna wasn't in the dining room. And she wasn't in the girls' house either. I didn't bother with dinner, didn't worry about a shower, went off caked in mud to find her, thought perhaps she might be at Piq. I turned right at the dead cow, starting to rot and smell more pungent with every day. Picked my way over rocks, over crushed roofs and walls, sighted a figure sitting down on one of the few intact houses. But it was Helen, not Anna. She was in need of peace, had no idea where Anna was, didn't even know she was missing, said the antibiotics for her womb infection were making her funny in the head.

I sat down next to her. We dangled legs, looked down the valley. The hyrax were underground, didn't come out until sunset. And we couldn't spot anything else.

So Helen turned and looked at me instead.

"I've been thinking about Christmas," she said. "I don't know what you and Anna are doing but I'd really like to spend some of it with you guys"

The day before, Anna had decided she would stay in Israel for Christmas and New Year. Her flight back was booked for Christmas Eve but she'd asked Marla to arrange one for the first week in January instead.

"That would be lovely," I said. "But we really want Christmas with just the two of us. I'm sorry. It might be the only Christmas we ever have together"

Helen understood. We returned our gaze down the valley. And then up she came, perfect timing to interrupt the awkwardness, pulling at grass and rock, root and sapling to help her back up through the valley. Her long black hair was tied back, away from eyes more distant than the Galilee behind her. I noticed bruises on her arms, asked where she got them from.

"Trying to knock down trees," she said.

Jimmy comes round with Arthur and Eleanor on their way to school, looks amazed when Anna steps out the door with the kids and I.

"When did you get out?"

"Last night," she says.

I'm further up when we enter the playground, trying to keep an eye on Joe and Arthur as they run ahead.

"How are things?" parents ask.

"Ask her yourself," I reply, nodding behind me.

They look on in admiration as she walks across the playground with Jimmy. Then the three of us walk back down the street again. For a few seconds I'm walking behind. I see the wind blow her trousers tight and wonder: has she lost that much weight already?

I hang the washing up in blustering wind. Blow a kiss to Anna through the kitchen window. She looks at the line, lets slip a wry smile. For once doesn't tell me how I've pegged it out all wrong. Then I come in, empty the dishwasher, feed Caffrey while Anna stirs flaxseed oil into cottage cheese, mentions how horrible it is, shows me homemade rhubarb crumble and home grown cabbage left on the doorstep by Lin. Radio 4 has a recorded interview with Jade Goody talking about cancer so I turn over to Radio 5. They have a phone-in about her. I manage twenty seconds, hear an outraged caller stating she had no dignity in death, switch it off.

Seaton Delaval Medical Centre provides the chance to continue our latest waiting room competition, started about two months ago. We pick up one celebrity magazine each. I have Heat and Anna has Hello; surely even odds. But it's me who finds a picture of Cheryl Cole first. And in a record time of just 2.4 seconds.

It's the first time I've seen her properly with no top on, more than just a peep down her neckline. The district nurse is taking her dressing off. Anna's lying on the bed, asks if I want to see her scar.

"I can see it from here," I say. But after a few seconds hesitation I inch closer.

"It's a very clean cut," says the nurse. "It will heal lovely"

The other nurse says nothing, has her hand on Anna's shoulder, her face contained. Doesn't want to look. It's like a little boy's chest; almost flat, no nipple. A little boy's chest on one side and a woman's on the other. But the little boy's side has been sliced from the middle all the way over and under her arm. It doesn't look gruesome or horrible though. It still looks like my girl lying there. And you won't have a clue when she's fully clothed, when she has her special bra with prosthesis. I wonder how many people I've walked past or spoken to have had their breast cut off, have had to go through the ordeal Anna has, that she'll have coming up.

Our team had their new strip on, looked all proud. Ricardo, Buchman and Guy played drums by the side of the pitch. Children waved flags and pom poms they'd made for the occasion. Eres' puppy dog gang ran onto the pitch and tried to get the ball off the players warming up. Afiq were playing an Israeli Arab team from a Druze village in the Galilee. But the opposition refused to turn up for political reasons. I'd arranged to go to Piq and watch the sunset with Rob after the match but walked to Bnei Yehuda with Anna instead. I knew Rob was sensitive about feeling left out and was upset I now spent most nights in the girls' volunteer house with Anna. But she was leaving in six weeks time and I wanted to spend as much time as possible with her. The next few days we worked together in the Avocado orchards, finished early, ate oranges and grapefruit from the trees, watched circling vultures and kept an eye out for a family of wild boar that had set up home there but would be shot dead within the week as they were considered dangerous. Those few days were among the happiest we spent there. We worked hard, climbed and picked trees, whistled and sang, chatted happily to each other and to the soldiers that worked alongside us. Ate huge breakfasts to fill ravenous stomachs. And my Mam had sent money from my Gran's will to a bank in Tiberius. So after work we planned to hitchhike there and have our first romantic meal together.

Anna takes pen and paper, tells Joe she wants to explain something. Draws a figure, adds two breasts and some hair.

"Now, you know Mammy went to hospital because she had a lump in her breast that needed to be removed?"

Joe nods, takes a bite of his cracker.

Anna draws a little round spot on the left breast.

"But that didn't quite work so the doctors thought it best just to take the whole breast off?"

Joe nods again.

Anna scribbles the breast out, does lots of dots all over the body.

"Well, our bodies are made up of billions and billions of little cells and the doctor wants to make sure that the bit that was bad hasn't spread somewhere else, where it would make another lump. So Mammy has to take really strong medicine"

She points at each of the dots with the nib of the pen.

"It's like hide and seek," she continues. "The medicine searches out any poorly bits and gets rid of them. That's good isn't it?"

Joe nods once more.

"And Mammy will have to go back to hospital to take this medicine. But only in the day time every three weeks and you'll be at school then anyway"

Pause...

"Oh, and there is one other thing"

"What's that?" asks Joe.

She shrugs.

"Well, the medicine is so strong my hair will fall out"

Joe looks quizzical, like he's trying to work out how medicine could make your hair fall out. But only for a second. Then he's back to crunching his cracker again.

Anna says she will have to go and choose a wig, tells Joe he can try it on if he wants.

Joe looks up, crumbs round his mouth, down his jumper.

"No thanks," he says. "It will be too big"

It was a stupid decision, a very stupid decision. And the ridiculous thing was; I had a sense of it at the time. And so did Anna, I'm sure. But we were tired and it was starting to get cold. And we so wanted to get back home. I climbed in the backseat, let Anna walk round the front. It took ages to hitch-hike to Tiberius in the first place. And so it was quarter to six and dark when we got there. And we didn't know which bank to go to because my Mam had been quoted a bank that didn't seem to exist. We tried two but by that time the rest were shut. Fortunately, Anna had a little money so we forgot about the meal, had a beer each, then walked to the edge of Tiberius to hitch-hike around the Sea of Galilee and back up the Golan. We'd waited three quarters of an hour before the car pulled up. And though my instinct told me it was a bad idea I chose not to listen. And so, even after I'd sloped my head down to the window and noticed two big men in the back and a driver in front, I still asked if they could take us to Afiq. The driver looked at us both and nodded. I didn't notice then if he looked at Anna more than me. I simply told Anna to get in the front, opened the back door for myself and squeezed in, shopping bag with vodka and cigarettes between my feet. The four of us sat in silence and watched Anna climb into the front passenger seat. Again, my instinct warned me, sent some kind of message shivering down my spine. But we were in, and the car was pulling off.

Round the corner of the Galilee we went, in silence, away from the lights of Tiberius, into the darkness of the countryside. Streetlights didn't exist in this part of the world, where settlements were few and the land had been stolen from Syria. A few words in Arabic were followed by a nod of the head. The driver leant across and touched Anna on the leg. I said nothing, kept quiet as my stomach crunched. Thirty seconds later he did the same but his hand lingered longer.

"Leave her alone," I said.

One of the men in the back answered me. He answered by leaning forward and placing his hand on Anna's bare shoulder.

"I would like to fuck your girl," said the driver.

"Stop it," I said.

The men kept touching her on the leg and the shoulder. The driver asked if he could fuck her again. Anna said nothing, sat still as a statue. The car continued around the Galilee in pitch black, me squashed to one side in the back, hand on the neck of the vodka bottle between my legs. Ready to fight when the car stopped but fully aware that each of these men were stronger than I was. And then the car turned away from the Galilee and headed upwards into the blackness of the Golan, kilometres before our usual turn off. My fingers gripped tighter on the bottle as the car drove upwards too fast for either of us to jump out, even if we could have telepathically told each other to. And the images of what was about to unfold became more and more horrific.

I placed my hand on the driver's shoulder.

"Let us out," I said. "Let us out." My voice raised. More desperate.

The car pulled off the road, slowed down over rougher track. I leaned forward and looked to the drivers mirror, stupidly hoping the fear in my eyes might be enough, might release some change in what was about to happen. But the darkness outside penetrated the car and smothered his features. I looked to the men on my left, my last hope of connection, of an opening to start pleading. But their faces were fixed firmly to the front, to where the car was headed. I swore to myself that I would fight to the death for my girl, that I would find inner rage from the depths of my soul. And yet my conscious mind told me I would have little chance. That two of these men could hold me while the other helped himself. Then the track dropped downwards and after two more minutes of silence we came back out at the Sea of Galilee. The car slowed down so we opened our doors. They pushed us out without stopping. I landed on the side of the road, my hands and elbows hitting dust. Anna fell into the middle. Up ahead the car stopped, turned around, then started our way again. I reached out and grabbed hold of Anna as it picked up speed. And then, as it passed us, a hand reached out from an opened window and grabbed hold of her sleeve. We were dragged along the road a few yards before falling to the ground once more. And then the car drove off into the darkness, while we hugged each other tight and sobbed.

I'm hanging out washing when Anna pops her head out, says Garfield is coming round for some coal. Can I fill a bag for him, take it round instead? Garfield is a friendly old feller who lives a few doors down on the other side of the road. He runs out of coal every few months, just for a couple of days or so but it heats all his water up as well as his house. Anna's told him he can come round anytime and help himself, get in through the back gate. I fill a bag up, walk across the road with it, wave at Kathy two doors down. Kathy is an old woman who lives alone. I've never talked to her and I don't think Anna has. I've never even seen her outside her front door. But whenever we walk down the pavement we see her through the window, sat in her big armchair, watching telly or knitting. Encouraged by their Mammy, Joe and Isla have always waved to Kathy every time they pass her house. She responds with a broad smile and sparkling eyes, a wave so exuberant it defies age. At Christmas they paint cards and pop them through her letter box. And on those occasions when they've been so excited they've jumped up and down laughing right in front of her very window Kathy's smile has reached epic proportions. I wonder what she thinks when she waves back, if she's simply taken by their beauty, innocence and childhood energy. Or if she's taken somewhere else, transported back to motherhood perhaps. Her own childhood. And when we walk further down the street does she continue with her happy memories? Or does her smile fade and die with the realisation she's sat in the same chair yet again? Knitting and watching telly as always. Garfield accepts the coal with a smile and a joke, tells me off for calling him 'mister.' Says he'll make some drop scones for us, bring them round later.

The district nurse peels back Anna's dressing ever so carefully. She's got an emergency appointment because of continued swelling underneath the wound, as if her body's protesting at not sporting a breast anymore. I move closer than I dared last time. The cut is jagged all the way across, purple and yellow bruise above and below. The nurse isn't sure what to do, thinks we should go back to the RVI for expert advice. Anna calls the ward but she can't go back. They're full. She was told that when she left earlier than the doctor recommended. So the nurse brings in the GP who tells her it looks infected and prescribes antibiotics.

I pick watercress and rocket growing in fish boxes we found washed up on the beach, make a salad. We eat it in the conservatory; watch our woodpigeon tenants on the trellis. They live in the conifer tree at the bottom of the garden, were there before we moved in six years ago. They start with foreplay, nibbling and pecking each other's necks in intimate fashion. Then it's onto full sex, which doesn't last long, before back to neck pecking. After two minutes of that, one shuffles away from the other. And they sit there for ages, not looking at each other, at opposite ends of the trellis. I stuff green leaves into my mouth, wonder if our pigeons are content, or if the one that moved away is in some kind of huff.

Anger rises through me. I want to cry and hit out at the same time. It takes me back to London, the Criminal Justice Bill protests, the ensuing riots I watched from close quarters. It makes me angry at this ridiculous world that's been created for us, enslaved in their money traps. For the first time in ten years I wish I was back in London, if only for the day. I wish I was part of this new protest at the banking system, at the way MP's used public money to claim all sorts of trivial and outrageous expenses. Then I drive past Joe's school and see all the pupils lined up. I make out Joe's blonde hair, Anna standing with other parents. A slow wave of warmth washes over me, casts anger aside. But I remember how Joe has these feelings of rage sometimes, of injustice. And how as parents we condemn that, try to iron it out, put it on the naughty step and take away treats. And I don't want him to lose that passion, that sense of injustice. And then I pull onto our drive and there's a rhubarb crumble and a pot of cream on the doorstep from Lin.

Anna's going back to bed. She went for a lie down after taking Joe to school, then got up for her salad. But her body's "wiped out," her head a "fuzzy mess." She's developed anaemia from the operation. The iron tablets and antibiotics are having an effect. Added to this she takes most of her painkillers at night-time, thinking awareness of pain during the day is probably not a bad thing, with the added advantage that painkillers at night knock her out a little and help her sleep. Well, that's the theory. Her wound feels further infected. I ask to see. Its swollen further, has continued growing, is almost half the size of her remaining breast. She phones her breast care worker, leaves a message, says anyone can call her back.

Some chocolate mini eggs and a card come through the letterbox. Then there's a knock at the door with flowers from Guernsey. I pat my tummy and estimate eight boxes of chocolate, two crumbles, three large cakes, one box of cup-cakes, two large chocolate bars, nine bunches of flowers, over twenty cards, two plants, two angels and a crystal in the past three weeks.

Anna goes back to the RVI to get her infected chest drained, comes back to flowers from Lin and the promise of another rhubarb crumble. Helen comes round and promises to do anything we want, brings flowers and chocolates from Ellen, an apology from herself for not baking.

The worst rain in Israel since 1956 and still they made us work. They had a contract to fulfil. Picked in all weather. The Golan was unrecognisable from when we arrived just two months earlier. By five a.m. twelve volunteers and soldiers were at the avocado orchards, freezing in waterproofs that weren't as effective as they should have been, trees and leaves saturated, ground clogged so thick with mud it almost reached Anna's knees in places. Within an hour we were soaked to the skin, finding it difficult to walk. Anna chose to work with Helen instead of me. I watched her as often as I could, examined her straightened face, wondered if it was just rain that streamed down her cheeks. When she returned my gaze guilt grabbed my face, twisted my head away. The weather seemed to wash most other issues away though. Songs were sung. Jokes were slung. And the laughter grew louder each time Helen fell because she couldn't lift her legs any longer. The tractor strugled more and more, got stuck in mud continuously. We had to group up behind and push it out, got splattered by scrambling wheels. Eventually the soldiers refused to work any longer and walked out, with Anna, Helen and myself following. Before we got back to the shed, Anna came into my arms in tears. Sometimes having time to think at work isn't such a good thing.

Anna's lying in bed trying to drift somewhere more pleasant than real life. I'm lying next to her with pen and paper, have just started scribbling when she pulls the duvet down, lifts her t-shirt up. The dressing's stained red from

111

the centre of her chest to her armpit. It needs changing and she needs me to do it. I follow her instructions. It's not difficult, simply a major plaster on a major cut. It trickles slowly this time, not like before on the bathroom floor. The t-shirt goes into a sink full of cold water. I take mine off and give it to her, then get back into bed as she goes downstairs to make a hot drink. My mind wanders to Tuesday. Results day. We'll find out how many lymph nodes are infected, if it's travelled into other parts of her body. How likely her chances of survival are. Whether that likelihood will drop further from 'good' and how far it will drop. How long she'll have left to live.

She comes into the bathroom as I'm drying myself from a shower. Her wound has continued to leak, her dressing stained red again. She places her second additional patch of the day over the swollen and leaking area.

"People will think I've had a reconstruction already," she says.

She won't go to the district nurse though. She'll keep patching it up until Tuesday. That side may be larger than her real breast by then but it needs an expert to look at it. And the district nurses don't have dressings big enough anyway.

I'm ironing a shirt, complaining about having to go back to work tomorrow, the usual Sunday night feeling.

Anna smiles.

"Yeah, but at least you don't have to go to work on Tuesday"

I raise eyebrows.

"Oh no, I'm going somewhere far more exciting"

Then she looks all serious.

"I haven't been thinking about it that much," she says, "not 'til today. And it's like I'm going to see a headmaster. Like I'm a naughty child about to get a report. Except this report is about life and death"

My mouth flattens. Speechless again.

"And I know they have the multi-agency meetings on a Friday. So I know the information's already out there, on how likely I am to live and how likely I am to die. And yet I don't know what it is. Won't find out for two more days"

Joe comes down to say he's finished his books, calls me a "fire-frog," goes back upstairs with his Mammy. Anna comes back down fifteen minutes later. As so often these days I smile but search her eyes at the same time. She realises I'm doing this, reaches up to the cupboard. I'm sure I see something but she slopes off to clean the toilet.

I start and finish a bottle of wine. Anna has a couple of tiny glasses but the rest is mine. We go to bed early, have nothing to say to each other. And there's nothing worth doing, not tonight. Half an hour after we put our heads down Anna sits up and peeks down her top. More blood is seeping through her dressings, all three of them. I get that sick feeling in my stomach. I can't cuddle her properly and don't see the point of praying. Surely at this stage it's just a matter of physics? Of tumour forcing itself through normal tissue. Slipping through walls of blood vessels. Hitching a ride in lymph fluid.

Isla's screaming, "I want my Mammy." I'm deep in dream, some absurd form of escapism. I stagger out of bed and stroke her head. She calms instantly. I imagine doing that every night, returning to a cold bed, waiting for my little girl to stir and scream once more.

The explosion arrived the same time as the flash. Or at least it seemed to. White light x-rayed inside and outside our house as it shook like it was collapsing into rubble. Rob was the only one standing up. He screamed, was knocked off his feet onto the couch. The lights and music went off. For a second I thought I was going to die as the bomb smashed the walls and roof on top of us. But stillness followed and the house remained intact. Anna came in, spoke first, said she'd been on the toilet, mumbled something about not wanting to die with her knickers round her ankles. Then we crept to the window and looked out as the storm raged all around us.

The banter, the tea-making, the photocopying and file-fetching, the frantic alarm collecting and register checking. But the welcoming smiles and thoughtful questions too, all about someone none of my work colleagues have actually met. Everyone's late this morning. We had to queue up and get sniffed by drugs dogs. All I could think about was tomorrow. Whether Joe's Mammy will live or disintegrate.

Whether Isla's Mammy will live or slowly crumble in front of her innocent colour changing eyes. And how the trauma will set them forever. But then it's time to move, and I'm lost in stories, in struggles with stories, in trying to move around the class and deal with practicalities such as pens and paper, files and notepads, what they're allowed to have and what they're not.

"How is your partner? Has she had the operation?"

"Yeah. It went as well as it could"

"Ah good, I'm sure she'll be fine now"

"She might not be"

"What?"

"She might not be. We get the results tomorrow. We get to find out if all of the removed breast tissue is cancerous or pre-cancerous. If it is then there might be more cancerous tissue left on her body. It might have spread further than they realised"

A look of blankness.

"And we get to find out how many of the lymph nodes they took out are infected as well. So far that one's fifty-fifty"

"No, no, I'm sure things will be fine"

Why do people do that? To reassure me or themselves? And then he tells me how his six year old niece died of bone cancer. How horrible it was for her parents to see her deteriorate.

I leave work and turn my mobile phone on to see if Anna's sent me a message. She hasn't. I've got three texts but they're all from friends. My novel has arrived through their letterboxes. They're really excited, can't wait to read it. It's not supposed to be out for eleven more days. I pick Isla up from Claire's, leave the car at our house because she hates getting a lift home, wants to run instead. We meet Annette on the way. She got my book on Friday, finished it today, says it's brilliant. We smile at each other while her daughter Heather pats Caffrey. And then we part on those lovely words, don't discuss what we both know is happening tomorrow.

Joe and Isla are in bed. And now Anna and I can't talk to each other again. I open another bottle of wine, order a curry. Joe comes down for a wee and a cuddle and then his Mammy takes his hand and leads him back upstairs. The wine doesn't taste good and the curry's too salty. We go into the back garden under bright shining stars. I fill up the bird feeders because Anna can't do it anymore. Still, we say nothing. We don't want to talk about tomorrow. And anything else would be completely irrelevant. So we go to bed and I cuddle in like a baby.

Maybe it was connected to the emotions of the last few days; the terrorist attack, the hitch-hiking incident, the kibbutz being struck by lightning. Perhaps it was my underlying despair that Anna would be packing her stuff, heading back to England, moving to Newcastle to start a new chapter in her life, because underneath our new found love we realised this separation could be a lifetime split, that it was likely we would both meet someone else sooner or later. Whatever it was, the images came first, weird and terrifying. I sat up in front of babies crawling in bin-liners, school masters laughing hysterically, dogs attacking each other, biting through flesh to the bone. Then the images faded to be replaced by a deep sense of being watched, observed by something or someone. The ceiling lifted away like a lid as I sat there, a tiny helpless animal in a cardboard box. I shivered, laid back down, covered myself in the duvet, inched towards the safety of Anna. But my eyes were forced upwards to the presence in the top right corner that looked down upon me. This was no ghostly figure or vision of any sense, but a feeling that was stronger and truer than sight. It neither hovered nor swooped, nor moved in any direction. It simply stayed where it was, whatever it was, and looked down upon me. Perhaps I said something for Anna was awake, holding my hand. But when I glanced across for reassurance she looked like no one I had ever met. And so my eyes returned upwards. They couldn't possibly go anywhere else. And I started to wonder: was this my Daddy looking over me? Was this my Daddy, his son in a strange and dangerous place, wanting to reassure me? And I became less frightened. My mind started to settle towards something resembling normality, though my heart rate still couldn't understand, still raced from all that madness. I made Anna put the light on and take me to the living room for coffee and hugs. She was there for me when I needed her, like I wasn't for her when she needed me. She held me and listened and I knew my Daddy would have approved of her, would have loved her. Warmed by Anna's hold I started to feel that this must have been my Daddy looking down, that he would be there to guide me through life, perhaps always was but had never needed to show himself before. A feeling of safeness heightened until it almost absorbed my whole body, until I was almost certain of the reason for all this. Yes, a tiny fraction wondered if I had contrived the interpretation because that was what I had wanted it to mean. But I dismissed this as devious tricks of the mind. We went back to the bedroom where images still came but faded after time. I told myself these later images must have been the result of my Daddy leaving, going back to wherever it was his energy and spirit lay, that the images that shocked me so much just an hour before were the result of him breaking through the barrier from his world to ours, a world he'd belonged to for just thirty years. And then Anna put her head down and tried to sleep. And he was gone from my life once more.

I lie still, then reach for my phone to check the time and she stirs. She sleeps so lightly these days. It only takes the slightest movement. But she keeps her eyes firmly closed and we stay that way, on our backs, faces to ceiling, for half an hour or longer, until the dawn chorus arrives. It stirs something in us, interrupts our frozen silence with moments of beauty. She tells me she hasn't slept a wink all night. I stroke her hair and look forward to the time when we can welcome the day like our feathered friends. Half an hour later I'm walking Caffrey down the street, dodging arched cats with spiked hackles. It's a gorgeous spring morning; blue skies and wispy clouds, joyous birdsong and warming sunshine. We reach the end of the street, continue over footpath. The tide is all the way in, has filled the harbour, lifted boats. A couple of fishermen are on board, getting ready to go off-shore. I walk around Rocky Island, wave to Kathryn. Then I help Joe and Isla get ready while Anna has a bath, makes sure her dressings stay dry. I help them wash their faces and brush their teeth, do a raspberry on their cheeks when they're finished, watch them run off screaming. It's impossible to understand how much love you can feel for children until you have them yourself, until you're in the same position. Until you watch them enter this world as helpless babies, grow into small children with character, humour and stubbornness, help them learn and understand. Until you feel childish yourself for being hurt when they snub you, in that undiplomatic and unwitting way only they can. All I have to do is look at them for a second or listen to them speak and I'm swollen with a pride and love I never knew I would be able to find.

I'm getting sick of this metro ride now. But at least this isn't the stifling and paranoid London tube. Newcastle's metro has a calmer atmosphere and runs mostly outside. Our carriage is full of sunshine, chatter and warmth. I read Anna her stars:

"You're getting a little too set in your ways as March draws to a close, Capricorn. You're reluctant to vary your routine and see anything new as an unwelcome intrusion. Loosen up a little"

She affords a wry smile as I search for mine:

"With the moon now in your own sign, March ends on a real high for you, Gemini. Confident, funny and very capable, you're in a league of your own at work. Here's hoping you can keep up the good work at home too"

Then it's Newcastle in the warm sun. We get out at Central

119

Station because we're early; all sunglasses, casual dress and shoulder bags. We could be tourists or mature students hanging around, enjoying the atmosphere, soaking up the rays. But we're on our way to Low Friar St, turning left up Clayton Street, looking for the wig shop. We find 'Natural Image' down a small side street, over the road from a Thai restaurant we went to years ago. A woman in her thirties meets us, smartly dressed and full of warmth, introduces herself as Liz. I look at her hair and wonder if it's a wig. Then we have a look around at all the different styles and colours hanging on the wall.

I pick one up with surprise

"Look, that's exactly like your hair is now"

Anna smiles.

"It is, isn't it? But I think I'd like something different for a change"

She needs time to try them on but we don't have it right now, so Anna promises to be back later if she feels up to it. We leave, agree we'll go for a meal at the Bangkok Cafe if there's any time left, play 'Spot the Wig' along the way. Past the Lebanese restaurant that does all day English Breakfasts. Around the side of the RVI to soak up the sun a little bit longer. Dodging smokers in dressing gowns getting ten minutes freedom, smoking themselves closer to death.

"If the news is bad," says Anna, "I'll probably refuse the chemo"

"You'll what?"

"If they give me six months to live, or a year, I'm not going to spend it zonked out with chemotherapy. I'm going to enjoy as much time as I can with my family, before I leave you all for good"

And then we're in the Leazes wing. And we've stopped speaking again, are just clenching each other's hands tight. Waiting room 5 is full, standing room only. The clinic's running an hour late. I count twenty-seven people and it seems only eight are supporting someone else. Anna has a quick chat with this woman she's seen at every appointment, from mammogram, tests and results, to surgery, more tests and more results. Then she picks up a magazine and I pick up a pen and look around. There's nobody her age, nobody as young. I look at them all and think at least you have children that have grown up, that can understand what's happening. That can fend for themselves and have probably left home already, have lives and families of their own. The surgeon comes out a small room, head lowered. I don't know anything about Dr Griffiths. I don't know if he has family, if he's lost anyone close to him. I've only met him three times and only then for ten minutes at most. I admire him greatly though, and I'm starting to feel extremely nervous about seeing him again. Names get called out; other people's. They go in, come back out again twenty minutes later. I've stopped glancing at their faces, trying to work out whether their news was good or bad. I just keep my head stuck in a magazine or paper. But every time a nurse comes out something inside of me jumps. And I feel more nervous, more sick. You don't want to hear her name, to have to stand up, walk past everyone else. But you need it to be over with. You've waited long enough.

And then they call her name. And it's our turn to go in....

PART V

It may not have been the greatest invention known to mankind, but it was the greatest invention known to Kibbutz Afiq volunteers in the winter of 1991. Sharon and I were understandably pleased with ourselves. And though excitement didn't quite reach fever pitch, everyone except Rob sampled the result and was delighted with the end product. And so subsequently, toast making on our new electric fires took off. Rob was away in Tiberius but a slice of bread was still placed on the fire guard and made for him. When he didn't materialise it was left in his Christmas stocking. And when he came back to the kibbutz during supper time and was told there was a present for him, he rushed back to the volunteer houses in anticipation. But when he stuffed his arm inside his stocking and pulled out a slice of cold toast he couldn't have been overjoyed because he came back looking rather sullen. Within a couple of days though, he began to understand how important this discovery was. Nobody had eaten toast for over two months. It seemed Israelis had not even considered the possibility. Soon, chocolate spread on toast followed mashed avocado and lemon juice on toast, and that recipe was improved by the cutting and rubbing of garlic. Within three days scrambled eggs were attempted, although this was not such a success. And within a week we were all given severe warnings about our behaviour, deemed to be a fire risk.

The nurse leads us inside, asks Anna to lie down. Says the doctor will arrive soon, check her wound, see how things are developing, let us know her results. Anna takes her top off and lies back. The nurse presses a lever to move the bed upwards. I sit on a chair at the foot of the bed and think, what is this for? It's irrelevant. We need results. We need to know if my girl is going to live, or if she's going to die from cancer like more than half a million other people in the past twelve months. That's what we're here for. Not a check on a wound for God's sake. Then Dr Griffiths comes in, calm and dignified as usual, gives nothing away. He sticks a needle through the wound, drains out blood and fluid, does it a second time. Then he goes to leave the room again, stops a moment and looks across at us.

"The nurse will take you through to another room where we'll go through the results"

We have to wait a few minutes first, have this room to ourselves. But as Dr Griffiths pointed us towards the door he let slip a clue, then wandered off for Anna's file. And now, at one of the most important moments of our lives, we're trying to decipher what he meant.

Anna's not sure what "favourable" means. She knows the word of course, but isn't sure how to put it into context. I tell her if you take the worst possible result and the best possible result, then draw a line right in the middle of those two, then surely "favourable" must be the best side of that. And then Dr Griffiths and the nurse are with us, bringing Anna's now bulging case file. He doesn't wait long, not this time, gets straight to the point. Last time he went through facts first, talked about what had happened for ten seconds before getting to the nitty gritty. This time he says it simple:

"None of your lymph nodes we took out during the mastectomy were found to be infected with cancer"

I see Anna breathe out. Feel her body go loose through the hand I've been holding tight.

"That's good news"

Dr Griffiths smiles, the nurse too. Anna joins them, then breathes out again.

"Oh, that's such a relief," she adds.

I ask how many lymph nodes there are under the arm and he says they took out thirty-something, then switches to the removed breast tissue.

"We didn't find any invasive cancer in the breast tissue," he continues. "There was in-situ cancer which would have developed into full cancer. We knew that though and that's why we went ahead with the mastectomy. But there wasn't any invasive cancer found"

Anna, the doctor and the nurse all know better than I how important these two statements are.

"Was there any healthy tissue in the removed breast?" Anna asks.

"There was some," says Dr Griffiths, giving the impression by the sound of his voice that this was little.

And so they discuss treatment with us. Chemotherapy for four or five months. After that, radiotherapy every day for three weeks. Tamoxifen and possibly Herceptin if she's found suitable for it. Then we walk silently through the waiting room, eyes glancing up at us, wait until we're in the corridor before we cuddle and kiss. I phone my Mam as soon as we're outside and her relief is evident. She asks if I'm okay, says I sound "tremulous." I tell her I'm fine, have been sleeping okay, that I have some ability to turn emotions off at times. She says men can do that, can sleep whatever is going on. Women lie awake at night worrying.

The day after Eres was thrown out of our house for eating Christmas decorations off the tree, we found Rob's missing flip flop half a mile away on the other side of the kibbutz. And although this surely wasn't the last straw, Rob made his mind up that he'd seen enough of Kibbutz Afiq and made plans to leave within the week. Before he left, Marla took the remaining six volunteers on her family trip to Gamla and Capernaum. I sat on the edge of a cliff with Rob, watched eagles glide at eye level, water cascade below in a rush of foam and noise. We didn't talk, just sat together as friends, in the knowledge that a girl had come between us, soured what could have been a great friendship. But I knew Rob would have chosen love if it had offered its warm hand. And I wondered if, like me, he had always secretly hoped it would, that it was part of his reason for leaving Britain in the first place. Marla, who was so kind most people thought of her as a mother, then took us to Capernaum where Jesus first started preaching and fed the five thousand on the shore of the Galilee. This time, we saw Peter the disciple's house. And then, wandering on rocks where Jesus held council, where he pushed his boat out to water, I discovered a hand grenade without its pin. Marla contacted the army. And we sat on the jetty and watched the sun go down.

Liz has been counting the hours, is pleased to hear our good news. Takes us to a private cubicle and after a brief chat ties Anna's long hair up inside a stocking and starts to bring wigs.

"This is the time to experiment. Try on some styles you wouldn't normally consider"

She brings the first one, ruffles it with fingers. Anna pulls a face. It's short and spiky and we both know it won't suit her. Still, Liz starts to lower it onto the top of her head. She looks ridiculous at first, like there's a small burrowing animal in between her head and the wig. Then Liz adjusts a strap and pushes it down further and it settles into the right place.

"How about this?" she asks. "This one's different"

Anna looks in the mirror, tips her head one way then another. Looks like she can't make up her mind. Like she may actually be considering it as a possibility.

Then her eyes glance my way through the mirror.

"What do you think?"

"You look like an Armenian prostitute," I say.

Anna giggles. Liz glares at me. I shrug. And then another wig is hovering above Anna's head, this one long with streaks in.

Down it goes, Anna hopeful once again.

"Spinal tap"

More giggles from Anna and another look from Liz. Neither of us care. We're giddy, high on the possibility of life. And Anna trusts my judgement. The next two are different though; they look the part. After five or ten seconds' adjustment, of both the wig and our eyes, they look good, natural even. We have a dialogue over which looks the best, can't agree. Anna decides to order one in another colour, make the decision when it's arrived. I ask Liz if they have any Rod Stewart wigs. It's not that type of shop she says. We say our goodbyes, go past the Bangkok Cafe, promise to eat there when we come back to buy the wig and try headscarves. I ask if we're still going to buy that campervan and she smiles and agrees. I ask her to marry me again too. But tomorrow we'll be alone and we'll plan the vegetable garden, do more planting and sowing, eat good food. Anna speaks to her brother after we put the kids to bed. She's shattered, doesn't have an appetite, just wants to go to bed herself.

"But it's like I can dare to dream of the future," she says.

The weather may have been the worst Israel had seen for over thirty years but it couldn't soak our love apart. Anna and I had a wonderful day picking the last of the avocados. We talked about Christmas, how we'd make the most of it, how it didn't matter if we couldn't afford to go anywhere because we had each other. When we got back to Afiq she went off to feed Uzi's dog. I got showered and changed and was wandering along to the dining room when Helen told me the news. There were no flights available in January, none whatsoever. Marla had checked. Anna would have to fly back Christmas Eve. She said Anna already knew, had received the news terribly then gone back to the house to find me. Christmas Eve was the following Tuesday. I went to find her, caught her walking back along the path, walked up and hugged her. She started crying. I didn't know what to say, was too shocked to talk. We hugged, walked in the cold, hugged and walked again. We'd accepted the fact that she had to go back to England. We'd accepted the fact our love might never flourish beyond the next few weeks; the cruelty of falling in love with someone on a different path. We'd accepted all of this instead of being despondent. All we'd asked was that we have a couple of weeks together, that we spend Christmas and the turn of the year together, that we put aside our heartache and enjoy each other. And then the New Year would come and bring whatever it thought right. But now even this had been snatched from us. Anna said if she couldn't change her flight she'd try and sell her ticket back to the airline, buy another. It was the only option we could think of. Her nursing was starting on the 9th of January. We gripped hands tight, pledged we would do absolutely anything to stop her going home before Christmas.

One of my most skilled abilities is to be able to flick boxer shorts up from the floor with my toe, get them to land on my head whilst naked and with both of my children throwing socks at me. Then, with voice raised, I tell Joe even Spiderman needs to wash his hands before breakfast. Downstairs, I ask Anna to show me her wound while she's cooking porridge. She pulls out her neckline, lets me look inside. Its bruised purple and yellow, still swollen, slightly oozing from one side. Two minutes later, Joe wipes porridge on his sleeve, tells Isla he's getting his level one swimming badge today.

Isla looks at his sleeve, pulls a face.

"Euurrgghh Joe, that's ingusting"

I pick up the kitchen compost bin, am about to take it outside to tip into the garden compost, then hesitate. I take the small notebook out my pocket, find two others and rip the pages I've already typed up into tiny little pieces, scatter them on top of the compost. I decide I will do this with everything I write. These recordings of suffering, of enduring, of dignity amongst difficulty; they'll help feed the soil and nourish our future.

I plant potatoes next to purple sprouting broccoli, transplant chives. Anna directs me. Then I pick some broccoli and we eat it with Lin's baby leeks and a tuna steak each. And we talk about the future like there really might be one.

I push Joe up the muddy slope, pull Isla behind me. Caffrey makes it no problem, reaches the top well before us three. We look at the view and smile, cup hands and shout to Anna back down below, walk through the archway of the small and almost completely ruined 18th century Starlight Castle. Sir Francis Blake Delaval was the man responsible, was said to have numerous lady dependents living in private houses on his estate near Delaval Hall. But when his latest addition arrived there was no suitable accommodation for her. He decided to build a castle for her but his friend, the actor Samuel Foote, burst out laughing and said castles couldn't be built in a day. Sir Francis won the hundred guinea bet by having sections of a tower prefabricated and teams of men working throughout the night so that it was built within twenty-four hours. Unfortunately it didn't last long and started to crumble. Meanwhile, Joe wants to walk along the top fields and come down near the bridge. I shout to Anna, tell her to meet us further along. She'd have come with us but was worried she might stumble. I get the feeling she's in a mood today. And staying at the bottom of the dene by herself won't have helped. She's used to joining in all adventures, initiating most of them. I guess the relief of clear lymph nodes has finally settled, the joy that followed, with the promise of life thereafter, evaporated. I imagine the reality of chemotherapy and radiotherapy and the years of drugs have all come back to press down heavily upon her.

What better way to start Sunday than strong black coffee in bed, cuddling children and Anna, followed by three successful flicks of boxer shorts onto head. After chants of "champion, champion", but only by me, I'm dressed quickly and out with Caffrey, Lin's homebrew rhubarb wine not affecting me in the slightest, which certainly couldn't be said about last night. I take Joe to Waves, the new leisure pool at Whitley Bay. Fountains, slides and a pirate ship with firing water cannons. Isla stays at home because children under five have to be accompanied by the same number of adults. I look around at the women, see all ages, all shapes and sizes. From young mothers to grandmothers. But I don't see any with one breast. I throw Joe into the air, listen to him scream, think how much Anna is missing out. She can't come here for six months. And then, when the chemo is over, when the wounds have healed, the risk of infection lessened, will she really be brave enough to overcome all those stares?

I have a new student in my creative writing class today; a muscular black lad with a gold tooth. He addresses me from the back of the class in his West Midlands Caribbean patois.

"I'm writing a book guv"

"Are you? What's it about?"

"It's an escape manual. How to get the fuck out of here"

"Ah right. What chapter are you up to?"

A pause, just enough for dramatic effect.

"The part where we take the teacher hostage"

Loads of laughter, myself included. I wait until it dies down.

"Right then, I'm just going to the toilet"

Another of my students is writing a poem to his best friend and wife. Their eight year old son was killed by a stolen car pursued by police. The funeral is on Thursday, the same day as my book launch. One of the most important events in my life and someone else's most horrific nightmare come true. We chat a little about this, how the extremes of life are all around us. He hopes the poem goes some way to reaching out to his friends, something it is physically impossible for him to do in person.

I'm dreaming my book launch has just finished. It was an outdoor event. Nirvana played. Thousands came, an amazing success. But the photographer and video man didn't turn up. Then I wake with a start and realise I haven't moved the time on my alarm clock one hour forwards. Instinctively though, my hand goes downwards. It's not just Anna's reading that's increased tenfold. I've checked my testicles more in the last two months than I have in the previous twenty-five years.

She talks about how easy it is to slip into patient mode. To put your life into the hands of others, even after so many years of being on the caring side. But it feels weird having to halt your life and watch everyone else carry on. She was out in Whitley Bay today. It made her feel a fraud, like she should be at work if she could go out shopping. She saw a colleague in the shopping centre, someone who's been off for months with stress. He was about to meet a team leader, was all tearful, looked like he was going to fall to pieces. Had a two week sick note with him, kept having to justify his absence. Anna had another three month sick note, no questions from anyone.

"That's how it goes," I say. "You can't argue with cancer"

My first thought, when I was able to navigate my brain through its pounding hangover, was "oh shit, we've missed the bus." My watch read five to five though. I woke Anna and Rob, dashed to the dining room to tell Denis the others were on their way. Denis took us to Kursi where we collapsed on the bus, still drunk but in surprisingly good spirits considering the importance of the occasion. I closed my eyes and recalled what I could of the previous night. We'd done our best to enjoy the Christmas party put on by Marla, cheered with everyone else at the Israelis who came along, including one dressed up as Santa. After the meal, an old American feller played the blues while we got drunk. Then we went to the pub at Bnei Yehuda and drank more.

I shook my headache, put a hand on Anna's knee, looked at Rob in the seat in front. He was staring out the window, saying a silent goodbye to the Golan. Was going to travel by himself for a few days, then fly home. I'd miss him for he'd been a great friend. But his leaving only forced me to consider how important the day was for Anna and I. We were going to Tel Aviv to somehow try and find a later flight. Anna said she was optimistic, felt something could be done, but as the outskirts of Tel Aviv came into view my nerves started to thump. Her eyes glazed over as the buildings drifted past. I closed mine tight and prayed. By nine a.m. we'd said emotional goodbyes to Rob at the airport. Then we explained what we wanted while this woman stared back at us, no inclination in her eyes as to whether our dream was possible, as to whether or not she understood how important it was. When we'd finished explaining she said there was one thing we might be able to do and one thing only. If that failed it meant Anna leaving on Christmas Eve, in three days time. Sometimes another company swapped flights. We went there and they refused point blank. And so back to the previous desk, but they wouldn't buy the ticket back however much we pleaded. We refused to leave so she phoned a few travel agents just out of politeness. If there was anyone behind us I'm sure she would have moved onto the next person, waved a hand at our protestations. Regardless, she didn't hold out any hope. The flights for cheap charters in early January were 220 dollars which was just about manageable if a company would be willing to buy her earlier flight. Two phone calls provided two negative answers. Our hearts sunk deeper than the sun we'd watched over the Galilee. She told us we would have to walk around the various companies and try them ourselves. The first had nothing but an indifferent shrug and a shake of the head. The second though, seemed more hopeful. We held hands and waited while he pressed keys and checked the screen. Then he looked up and smiled. January 8th was available for 196 dollars, including exit tax. Our tears said all the thanks necessary. It was all the money she had but it didn't matter. We went to the beach, hugged arms around each other, paddled and found shells, sunbathed because the weather turned from rain into bright sunshine especially for us.

In comes Dave's text: "Houston we have lift off." I open it up and there's a picture of me in the Northern Echo, a full page write up. After a family trip to the dentist where Isla refuses to sit in the 'up and down chair' but manages to get two fairy stickers just for opening her mouth, I deposit the rest of the family to go and buy wine for tomorrow's launch. A quick in the car phone interview with the Hartlepool Mail, the town of my childhood and teenage years, a chat with the publisher who tells me nobody will be able to come up for my launch, and I'm struggling on the metro with twelve bottles of wine and five bottles of mineral water. My arms feel like they're going to pull from their sockets. And I'm thinking to myself, I'd never dreamt it this way.

Anna's at Helen's, trying on dresses and tops. She wanted to buy something new for the book launch but hasn't had the time, wants to look good on the night. It's important. She wants me to feel proud of her. But she's got to be careful about what she wears. Nothing too low cut and nothing too hot in case she needs to take it off.

Lying in my bed around ten, I've a knot in my stomach. I had a look around Waterstone's today, a chat with Kristine, the events manager. Met Dawn, my lovely artistic friend, for lunch. I didn't spend too long on the computer after the kids went to bed. Didn't want to get involved in facebook or e-mail conversations that would keep me up too long. And so I'm lying here, in bed with this tightening knot, feeling nervous about the growing realisation there may be a large crowd tomorrow. And yet I realise it's stupid considering other things that are going on in our lives right now. Considering the last two months, the year ahead. All I've got to do is stand up and read a few lines, sign some copies of books and appreciate friends and loved ones.

I'm here before anyone else; just a few browsers looking at poetry, foreign language, with no idea and probably no interest in what will be happening in forty minutes. And the thing that strikes me most, apart from the fact I seem to be getting calmer rather than more nervous, is how small a display one hundred books makes. I wander around, look at empty wine glasses and full bottles, let disappointment seep in that nobody from my publishers made it up from the London-centric literary world. John and Sean are the first to arrive, coming up stairs to quiet handshakes and empty surroundings. The next is Alan, a manager in Sunderland Youth Offending Service and ex-training colleague. Half an hour later the place is crammed and the events manager looks nervous. And I realise I'd better do something.

After our good news at the airport, even cleaning chair legs in the dining room was fun. We listened to Nick Cave and

Led Zeppelin, tided our rooms afterwards we were in such good moods, went for the Shabbat meal then fell asleep. It was half past midnight when we woke up but we still went to the pub. It was the Golani's last Friday night before the older ones left the following week. They were all there; both Hanan's, Duron, Sharon, Decker, skinny Yossi, Alle, Uzi, Amit, all of them. Jumping up and down, laughing, getting drunk, talking to everyone and taking photos. All except a couple who didn't know what to do with themselves, who looked as if they were going to burst into tears. None of them knew what they were going to do afterwards and most of them were scared and nervous beneath that Goldstar beer exterior. Twenty-one or twenty-two and not one of them had led a life of their own. Straight from school and straight into the army. So wise and aged in one way but so naive in another and they knew it. When the pub finished Anna and I stole some half finished wine bottles, took them back to the lads house and spent the night there, feeling the absence of Rob and the coming of a new moon for so many who'd been stuck on top of the Golan the last few months. We stayed in bed all the next day, took back food from the kitchens, the kettle from the girls house, finished the wine, earned the nicknames John and Yoko. Shirley and Sharon came in and told us they were going to Jerusalem for Christmas, were really excited because they hadn't been there yet. Anna spoke with so much enthusiasm and zest I found it a struggle not to laugh. She told them how incredible it was, how lucky they were to be going, especially at such a time. I had to leave the room because I couldn't contain myself. I went to Denis to arrange my secret plan. He agreed to put us both on the work list for the 23rd. I asked for the avocados, as that meant getting up the earliest.

I wake full of energy, jump up and dance in my boxer shorts. Anna smiles, then groans and turns over. I continue dancing. I don't need an audience, not today, not this morning. Granted, I'm still drunk and that might have something to do with it, but it's not the whole story. I read Isla's story as fast as I can then the kids are jumping on me and I'm throwing them off and Anna's decided it's safer and calmer elsewhere. And I'm up again, dancing and singing once more, flicking my boxer shorts on my head, Joe and Isla screaming with laughter, bouncing on the bed. And I want to do it all again. I want to tell the world, read them the story of Danny, the sixteen year old you'd want to cuff around the head and take home to adopt all in one go.

The books sold out. There weren't enough copies. People were left holding thin air, disappointed looks on their faces. Myself and Rick Fury, the brilliant young rapper I performed with, only had time for two readings. The book signing queue afterwards took over half an hour. People got to the front of the queue, kept asking if my wrist was aching. I could have signed another hundred, another thousand. I felt like a bridegroom surrounded by people I love, by colleagues and ex-colleagues, people I didn't know invited by others as well. Anna looked fantastic, everyone said, knew as many people there as I did. I take champagne out the gift bag, open cards I'll keep forever. There wasn't enough time to get round everyone, to give them my thanks. There were just moments and movement, then alcohol.

I breathe in deep, put a hand to my side. Wonder if I'm starting to feel hung-over...

On the beach with friends, that's the way to clear the head and stomach, with Wej and his two beautiful girls Izzy and Elysia. Trousers, socks and shoes off, sandcastles and spinning round in circles. We charge the sea shouting, run away screaming. Tread shattered fragments of sea coal and midnight blue shells further into sand. Then it's back to reality, reading books to my children at bed time. It's my turn to read to Joe tonight, a chapter of The Enchanted Wood followed by Horrid Henry and the Mummy's Curse. A boy with a love of stories already sewn into his soul. And then it's six in the morning, and reading is how we start the day as well as finish it, and Joe wants me to read another Horrid Henry story, shouts "it's not fair" when I tell him I can't read the whole thing. Stamps his feet on the ground, fails to see the irony of it; how he sounds exactly like Henry himself.

We leave with hugs, homemade flapjack and eggs from their chickens. Over the Weardale Valley we go, past startled pheasants and delicate spring lambs, curving and dipping through heather as life springs back after frozen winter.

There's something about those wisps of golden curl, those searching eyes that turn to sparkle. They take it in turns coming into our arms. Hug like they really do know how important and healing it can be. My sister's girls are magical; Jasmine aged six, four year old twins Rosie and Lily, the most loving and tactile children I've ever known. We eat great food outside their house, watch five children between the ages of three and six run about, swing through the air 'til their toes point upwards, their hair falls backwards. I join them for ring a ring of roses on the trampoline before they climb up Mike's camouflage spy tower. Then we walk down the stream to collect crystals for our garden and vegetable path. WH Auden said it was in Rookhope that he first became aware of himself as a poet. Perhaps he saw poetry in the collapse of lead prices in the late 19th century that caused many local mines to cease production, many men to lose their jobs. The demand for fluorite in modern steel-making gave a reprieve to many of the mines. Who knows; perhaps Auden helped himself to some of it too. But the collapse of the British steel industry in the early 1980's put an end to large scale commercial mining in Weardale, as it did in the rest of the UK. People's stories slip further back into folklore. We slip down the bank, fill a large basket, heave larger encrusted rocks up to the top and push them along in a wheelbarrow. Anna sits and rests as the kids run up to the top of the hill, play in long grass. Someone walks past, gives us a look. Rachael says something about mining rights, how somebody will own the crystals we're taking. I tell her it's a public place, is part of nature. But the rocks are so heavy we decide we can't take them all this time. And so on we go, through what WH Auden described as "the most wonderfully desolate of all the dales," chugging up small lanes as the day fades away, in our old Volvo laden with crystals.

The alarm went off at quarter to five. I let Anna lie in bed and moan for half an hour. Then asked her to read a letter. She didn't understand, said we'd better get up. I insisted. She read slowly, seemed too surprised to show emotion, then called me a bastard for making her think she was working all Christmas and hugged me. Said it was the best Christmas present she'd ever had. Denis had played along the day before, told Anna there was a picking in the orchards and he expected everyone to work harder than ever. But now Anna knew the truth, she couldn't go back to sleep she was so excited. We got up and had breakfast, packed in a hurry of excitement. After an hour waiting for a lift Marla took us to Zemach where we caught a bus to Jerusalem. Only then did I realise I should have planned ahead more than simply surprising Anna. Christmas in Jerusalem would be heaving with people surely? We rushed to the Faisal Hostel and were lucky. Ali recognised us, hugged and kissed us, showed us a double mattress on the floor, said we had to share it with an Australian girl. The hostel was packed. People who'd never met sharing beds, others sleeping under tables in the corridor. We went and sat on the balcony, watched the comings and goings at Damascus Gate, heard the call to prayer boom from speakers so loud it was as if it came from the sky itself. The Buddhist monk was still there, the old American and English eccentrics, the writer from Time Magazine too. Three cowboys walked in with all the gear, frowned when I said "Howdy" to them. We went for a walk in the dark, skirted around the Old City wall, came back and said goodnight to the Australian girl who looked embarrassed to be sharing the same mattress. Fell asleep sometime after midnight. The next day was Christmas Eve. We visited Yad Vashem, the museum and gardens in memory of the six million Jewish victims of the holocaust, given its name from the verse of Isaiah: "And to them will I give my house and within my walls a memorial and a name (Yad Vashem) that shall not be cut off." We walked past sculptures of twisted bodies caught in barbed wire, of babies clinging to mothers, photographs of people slumped on dirt, of death camps and ghettoes. Smiling families lining up for a train, overlaid with the sound of marching feet and screams. We read tales of survival and hope, discovered piles of shoes and glasses. And at the end of a long corridor, we found a large room filled with lights and the names of thousands of children; the whisper of innocent souls.

On the night we went to a candlelit midnight mass in the Old City, at the Lutheran Church of the Redeemer. The mass was in Arabic, German, Danish and English and finished just after half eleven. We stayed by ourselves in the church until after midnight, held hands but didn't speak. Sent prayers to all our loved ones back in England and in Israel. Then we went outside and joined the carol singing in a beautiful two tiered courtyard.

I'm walking Caffrey around the harbour in a sleepy early morning stagger when Billy's Dad approaches, hand outstretched.

"Here," he says. "Something to give your bairns for Easter"

I take the plastic bag, notice a claw sticking through the side.

"Are you sure?"

"Well aye. Put them in the bath or something. Tell them they didn't have any chocolate eggs left in the shop"

I buy the Sunday papers, dump them in the kitchen, go upstairs to find the children. They stand fascinated at the sight of two huge crabs, claws and legs moving around, large pincer slowly opening and shutting. Antennae zooming back and forth like a race that keeps finishing and starting again. I take them downstairs, tie the top of the bag, put them outside and boil the kettle. Look through the window and watch the bag slowly moving. Then I turn the computer on to help, have never done this before. I'm fine cooking dead things, preparing them even. Richard brought us pheasants. We plucked them together, cooked them separately, came together for a meal. He's hoping to bring duck or rabbit next. Chris and Katherine bring us twenty-odd mackerel every year, straight from the sea. But this is different. They're alive and moving. And although that's hypocritical and this bit's quite possibly pathetic, the sad truth is I'm more worried about one of them nipping me than the thought of boiling alive one of earth's creatures. I get two large pans of water bubbling, check the internet to make sure I'm doing things properly. Anna comes in, says she doesn't want to be cooking the kids porridge when I put the crabs in boiling water, when they start to squeal. I'm more concerned with how I'm going to get them into the pans. My first idea was to put on a gardening glove and hold the bag upside down so they drop in, but that doesn't seem practical. How can I get just one to fall into each pan? And Anna says I can't use gardening gloves anyway; it's unhygienic. So I put a marigold on, an oven glove over the top, reach into the bag and eventually pick one up by its back legs. There was a more humane way suggested on the internet, which included stroking the top of the crab's head until it fell asleep first. But I didn't fancy my chances with that one. I dangle it over the pot. Anna calls it torture but she's fascinated. I wait for the water to boil rapidly then lower it down, repeat with the next one. Wait for squealing but don't hear any.

Anna's losing her temper. She's sick of repeating herself. Sick of nobody listening. Sick of children refusing to brush teeth. Sick of Isla refusing to wear any knickers or trousers. Sick of me scribbling about crabs and crystals while she encourages kids time and time again.

We walked hand in hand, cajoled and joked, cuddled and cantered past elephants, hippos, wolves and monkeys. We followed peacocks that roamed free, waited for a feather to fall out but none did. The biblical zoo was all ours that Christmas day. We didn't see another soul as we wandered around. Then we got the wrong bus back and ended up miles away, eventually got back to the hostel at eight p.m. Met a conservative looking middle aged Australian woman who'd danced naked with aborigines, built and sailed her own boat, travelled around much of Africa and taken most drugs imaginable. She gave Anna a bracelet from Kenya as a Christmas present, said she wished she had something for me. We sat up drinking vodka with new friends for the night; Angus from South Africa, Melissa from New Zealand and an English feller called James. When the girls crashed out, Angus told me I should visit Ein Yahav after Anna left. Said it was the biggest moshav in Israel and there would definitely be work. I'd get paid more than the kibbutz's token one pound per day, would be able to save up for more travelling. The next day, Boxing Day morning, I woke up early, wandered outside to find two Shalom Peace posters we'd spotted the other day. I wanted to buy us one each, wanted us to have something exactly the same when we parted, something we could look up at in our own rooms, a picture that symbolised our time together. Up towards Jaffa Gate I staggered, in a half drunken daze, smiling to myself at where I was. I bought the posters but they cost eight shekels each because the owner refused to barter. Then we hugged Ali and the others goodbye and got the bus back up north. Anna fell quiet as we left Jerusalem behind. We didn't speak for hours, just looked out the window as our new home and life turned its final pages. I dreamed of further adventures but my heart churned at the thought of saying goodbye. Then we arrived back at Afiq after getting a hitch all the way back from Tiberius. And we made love and gripped each other as tight as we could.

Joe's absorbed in his Spiderman annual when his Mammy interrupts.

"What does this look like?"

But the Green Goblin's about to launch an attack.

"Joe!"

He looks up from Natural Image's comfy couch.

"What does this wig look like?"

He looks her up and down, no recognition in his face.

"Strange," he says, before returning to more important issues.

Anna chooses the wig that looks the least odd. Somehow, they don't seem quite so natural today. Then we get a headscarf, three English Breakfasts and some trainers for Joe, who dismisses all our suggestions and is only interested in trainers that flash or have hidden Transformers in their heels.

Isla's got the spanner, Joe the screwdriver. Building Grandad has got the know-how and I'm lying on my back trying to thread the screw. Within ten minutes we're lifting it over the little pond, standing back and admiring. But still Joe and Isla aren't allowed on. Ribbon is fetched, scissors from the kitchen, the camera's dead battery replaced. The garden is starting to look beautiful again. Honesty, tulips, primulas, daffodils, hyacinth, hellebores, lilies and hebe all encouraged by Anna and the great spring we've had so far. And then Building Grandad's bridge, made with two IKEA bedsteads, is officially declared open amid clapping, laughter and the clicking of photography. Joe and Isla walk on from opposite sides, wave at the audience of four and agree to cuddle in the middle for a photo opportunity.

This week's donations are as follows:

Small Easter cakes, a large apple cake, four cans of Guinness and two bottles of homemade rhubarb wine from Lin

Cauliflower seedlings and onion sets from Les

Easter eggs from Arthur and Eleanor

Easter Eggs from their nana Ellen

A big box of biscuits from Sandy and Jerry

A carrier bag of sweets and chocolate from Noelene

Gingerbread Easter bunnies from Building Granny and Grandad

Homemade flapjack from Rachael

A big bag of revels, a big bag of toffee popcorn and two big bars of chocolate from Judith

I open the biscuits and wonder how I'm ever going to get fit at this rate.

But Joe's noticed something he wasn't aware of beforehand.

"Daddy, what's that Ben 10 thing up there?"

He climbs onto the stool, puts his hands on the fridge. Looks around for some sort of grappling hook.

"It's mine," I tell him. "It's my Easter egg from your Mammy"

"What? That's not fair. I didn't get a Ben 10 Easter egg"

"I know mate but you did get lots of others"

He looks disappointed. The truth is that it was bought for him. But Anna decided the kids had too many already and so didn't give them ours. That's when I persuaded her I would make a worthwhile recipient instead.

He complains some more.

"I'll swap if you want Joe"

"What?"

"I'll swap you"

And so his face lights up as he gives me a much bigger smarties egg in return.

I held onto a branch with one arm, wiped rain from my face with the other, squinted and looked at my watch. Half five on New Year's Day morning and I was high up a tree in the pouring rain. Then the wind picked up and I hung on for dear life while cold water rushed down my neck and Anna grinned on the other side of the trunk. New Year's Eve hadn't been the stoned twenty-four hour John and Yoko love-in we'd dreamt about. We'd picked avocadoes all day, fallen asleep until half eleven, ran to the pub as fast as we could so we'd feel at least a little bit tipsy before midnight. But they only had one beer left so we had to share it. Helen was despondent, was missing Uzi, was going to miss Anna and I, other kibbutzniks and soldiers she'd lived with for the last three and a half months. Was worried about her upcoming operation as well. The Golani were only staying until March, but most of the older soldiers, including Uzi, had already left. Anna and I weren't thinking about leaving, were simply delighted to have spent Christmas and New Year together. We climbed the highest avocado tree we'd ever seen, got stuck at the top, giggled to each other, worried about climbing down wet branches. Anna went first, landed in mud at the bottom. I stayed where I was, looked across the tops of trees, to the mountains of Jordan and Syria. I had no idea what the new year would bring or where it would lead me. And though I'd done my best to convince Anna she was doing the right thing by studying to be a nurse back in England, I desperately wanted her to stay with me, to join me on my adventures wherever they would take me.

Anna sits on the rocking horse as she explains, her leg swinging round and round in a circle. After two or three minutes, it stops and goes round the other way. She's been for her pre-chemotherapy assessment at North Tyneside General Hospital, is getting a central line tunnelled under her skin, threaded into a large vein in her chest.

"What the hell's a central line?" I ask.

"A long hollow tube made from silicone rubber. They're going to pump the drugs into me through it. It's easier than injecting because it stays in my body the whole four months"

"Bloody hell"

"Yeah I know. But injections can lead to collapsed veins, and because all my lymph nodes have been taken out I can't have injections in my left arm"

She says the risk of infection is much higher than usual and she has to go straight to Accident and Emergency if she's worried about anything. If she gets an infection she'll have antibiotics pumped into her body using the same line, which also needs to get flushed once a week. I eat some more chocolate cake and ask how she feels about it. She says surgery was the easy part. She needs to rest every day, even if she doesn't feel tired. The main effect will be having no energy whatsoever, the "lead boots." Chemotherapy destroys weak cells but it also destroys white blood cells too, and these are the cells that fight infections so she'll be particularly vulnerable to everything. Even colds are really serious. She's been given a list of non-consumable items as well, can't have soft cheese, pro-biotic yoghurts, any antioxidants like green tea. They interfere with treatment. She's been given special toothpaste, toothbrush and mouthwash.

"I tried the wig on today," she adds. "But I only kept it on fifteen minutes because it felt really uncomfortable"

I glance behind her and there it is; hanging high above the telly on a piece of driftwood.

"Do you know when the chemo's starting yet?"

"Next Thursday," she says. "Six sessions. One every three weeks. As long as I don't get an infection because that'll knock things backwards"

I finish my chocolate cake, all the while watching her. Tell myself I need to get healthier, for everyone's sake. Her eyes turn inwards for a few seconds, then focus back on me.

"My hair's going to start coming out after the first session," she says.

She's never told me she's scared, not once. She's never even said she's nervous. She just looks at me with doleful eyes when I tell her I love her, that I'll always love her. I go over on computer chair wheels, realise she's quite a bit higher sat up on the rocking horse. I put my head on her lap and she rubs my hair while I sneeze, feel a cold coming on.

Down the dene we go, checking for caves, secret paths. Putting heads into tree hollows to say hello to animals, promises of picnics in the months to follow. I try to photograph sandpipers and lapwings, fail time and time again as they curve away with a shriek, glide upwards as if my camera were a gun. They circle around me. I spin in frustration, unable to capture them in my sights as an old chuntering crow mocks loudly. We arrive back to a pile on the doorstep, some books for the children, a rhubarb crumble, fridge magnets and a large smoothie.

I bring my arm back, throw the ball, knock four out of six tin cans over. Then notice the sign that says you have to knock them right off the plate. No wonder it seemed so easy. The second ball leaves just two lying on their side but the crucial third misses completely. Isla looks disappointed. The man gives me this stupid wiggly thing on a stick instead of a three foot cuddly gorilla. Another two pounds, another failure and Joe has a wiggly thing on a stick too. The funfair's quiet, cold wind and grey clouds ensuring last week's excitement has already blown over. Then, chastised by my failure on the tin can range, I choose the easy option instead and march over to hook a duck. Within two minutes I've won Joe a plastic gladiator sword and Isla a plastic hairdryer kit. Helter skelter, bouncy castles, slides, dodgems and a gentle rollercoaster lighten their moods further, as well as our pockets. The sword and hairdryer are both broken before we get home. Then, when Isla and I get back from the fish and chip shop, Anna's sat at the table with her wig on, looking rather obvious and not looking me in the eye. We tuck into our food. Joe, who's already glanced up at his Mammy a few times between mouthfuls of chips, asks her if she has a wig on. No, she says, continuing to eat and continuing not to look at me. Perhaps she knows what I'm thinking. I'm tired and irritable and looking at Anna in that wig that sits on top of her head like a sleeping animal only serves to increase my irritation. And then her eyes meet mine and she rolls hers upwards as it to acknowledge my thoughts. Fifteen minutes later she takes it off.

"Is that a wig Mammy?" asks Isla, noticing for the first time.

"Yes darling"

"Can I try it on Mammy?"

"Of course you can. Finish your fish and chips and then wipe your hands because they're messy. Then you can"

But she refuses to wipe her hands properly so the wig isn't passed onto her, however much she groans.

Yossi was the coolest Israeli I ever met, a good friend too. But he wasn't himself that morning in the dining room, said the kibbutzniks had called a meeting. He was being evicted, had to leave the next day. We put our cleaning cloths on the table and sat down. He cried, said every time he went back home he had fist fights with his father. Then, whenever he was at Afiq he needed to be alone and so walked out of work constantly. I had lunch with him, collected some food for Helen who was sick. I didn't notice the sky was unusually heavy when I stepped outside. Just carried on walking, swinging Helen's food in a bag.

The first snowflake I noticed was the one that landed on my hand. I watched it melt on my warm skin, saw others come down to join it. Within minutes it had turned into a blizzard that lasted two hours. The kibbutz went berserk; there was no other word for it. For many of them, it was the first time they'd ever seen snow. Ricardo, head of the kitchens, climbed onto the roof to take pictures. Soldiers ran around screaming, taking part in joyful and chaotic snowball fights. Itsic, working in the laundry, ran outside every five minutes, threw snowballs and jumped up and down. The transformation was incredible. I had never met a group of people more serious in my life. I'd had numerous conversations where I'd been told the holocaust could happen again anytime, at any given moment. We were surrounded by barbed wire, by patrolling army units. We were living on one of the most hotly disputed pieces of land in history. And here, all around me, grown men and women were squealing with delight, swinging their arms like five year olds because the clouds above were emptying snow upon them. The feeling was infectious. I rolled snowballs and hurled them at soldiers, took one on the side of the head to everyone's delight. But then I looked up at the dining room window and noticed Yossi looking out, all alone. He thought he'd be spending the next three years with Itsic, with Gillie and the rest of his friends. He'd invested his future, his emotions, his life to these people as they approached three years national service together. He had a girlfriend at Afiq too. But he was leaving tomorrow, whether he liked it or not. Anna and I went round to the Bronx to find his home later that night. We chatted for hours. Nobody else went round to see him. I gave him Neil Young, Lou Reed and The Cure. He gave me Velvet Underground and Siouxsie and the Banshees Live in Tel Aviv. We played the Banshees tape all the way through. When they came back on for their encore and played 'Israel,' the reception made hairs all over my body stand up like wire. And then we hugged a final goodbye.

After Isla and Joe have tickled Aunty Judith to a frenzy, we drive to Granny Annie's and Grandad Barrie's. And for the first time in twenty years, who knows maybe thirty, the chicken leg goes to someone else. My Dad has one as usual, but the other goes on Anna's plate. People talk about loss of appetite and Anna's mentioned it a few times. But she's polishing off a large plate of chicken, roast potatoes, salad and coleslaw and when asked if she wants custard or cream on her pudding replies with the customary "both." I wonder how things will change once chemotherapy starts. My Mam's already ahead of the game, gives Anna turmeric root and apricot kernels, says turmeric is a wonder spice that can prevent cancer among many other benefits. Apricot kernels are more controversial though. They're the seed from inside the apricot stone and are the planet's richest source of Vitamin B17, one of nature's most powerful anti-oxidants. But they also contain cyanide, which gives them their bitter taste. Our healthy cells have an enzyme that helps protect them from the cyanide, but cancer cells don't have the enzyme and so get zapped. You should take ten each day for the prevention of cancer and forty for treatment. That's one side of the argument; the side my mother takes, and others who complain medical research has a billion dollar cancer industry to support. The other side states they're highly toxic, highly dangerous. The Food Standards Agency recommends no more than two a day. I ask Anna if she's going to take them but she won't give me an answer.

There's a comfort in patterns, even when they're not constructive. Even when they're boring and stale on occasions. Our pattern was set a while ago: put the kids to bed, tidy up and then I jump in the computer chair as soon as possible whilst Anna potters in the garden if it's light enough and in the house if it isn't. Then Anna gets a shower and I walk Caffrey and we both get into bed to read a little and sleep. This time though, I go outside and Anna has me emptying compost into fish boxes. Breaking patterns can be refreshing, can open up chinks of light. We go to bed early, hold hands, play with each other's fingers. Look up at the ceiling. Eventually it's me who breaks the silence.

"Are you alright?"

It feels like a stupid question as soon as it leaves my lips.

But she smiles.

"Yeah"

I look deeper.

"Yes but are you *really* alright? Or are you just pretending you are?"

She removes her attention from the ceiling, looks across at me with watery eyes.

"There's times I'm dreading the chemo. Of course there is. I feel like just cutting my hair off straight away. It's stupid really. But I'm alright now. I'm in an okay place"

Then she looks at the curtains and carries on.

"I just hope the kids are going to be okay, that they won't be messed around too much. Farmed out all the time"

"They'll be fine," I say. "Isla wakes up every morning with 'Where am I going today?' She's independent. She wants to go places"

"She's changed," says Anna, "since I've been to hospital the twice. She never used to be clingy when I left her and now she is every time. I'm worried she'll struggle at school"

"She's at a crossroads," I say. "Claire twice a week, nursery once a week. It hasn't been enough for her to settle and that's not helped. That and knowing she's starting school soon. It's bound to be unsettling for her. She'll be fine when she gets going every day. And it's only a couple of hours to begin with. What you're going to go through might have hardly any effect on the kids whatsoever"

She doesn't answer, just continues looking at the curtains. I stretch my arm out, turn the light off. And we lay there in dark silence.

Anna's Mum wants to take her to the first chemotherapy session. I was taking her until it changed to Thursday. Anna wants to go alone though, is insisting upon it, says everyone who works there is lovely, Louise is bringing her home. She's asked her Mum to pick Joe and Isla up from school instead. But I feel as if I'm letting her down and I bet her Mum does too. Until last week her chemo was Wednesday, my day off. But they've decided to put the central line in then instead. I said I'd take the day off but Anna said she'd rather I went to work. And I just accepted, didn't even argue, probably because I've had so much time off work recently. The prisoners ask how she's doing on a regular basis. I told them she was going for the operation because I didn't want them thinking I was slinking off lots without valid reasons. Plus, they knew I was writing things down because we talk about the therapeutic nature of creative writing regularly. They all said if she needs looking after I should drop them like a stone and go to her side. Anna says she'll be okay, for at least six hours after anyway. It's the following days she'll need help, when she gets sickness, pain and exhaustion.

We heaved our rucksacks on the six-thirty a.m. bus to Tel Aviv, dumped them on seats in front. People stared as we touched each other's faces, held hands and stroked legs. We stared back, defiant. But only for a few seconds before our attention turned to each other again. Helen had left the day before without saying goodbye, said she'd be too emotional, had cried and hugged us the day before that. Our final night was spent packing rucksacks in separate houses as most of Anna's belongings were still over at the girls' house, though we popped across to see each other frequently. I wrote a note and secreted it in her rucksack. She sat on my knee, gave me her Peter Tosh tape, the greatest cuddle ever.

When we arrived in Tel Aviv we got a taxi to the nearest hostel, dumped our rucksacks and bussed it to Jaffa, one of the oldest port cities in the world, built by Japheth, Noah's son, after the flood. We walked along the promenade hand in hand, climbed up under minarets and palm trees to a commanding view of the Mediterranean, of Andromeda's Rock, where a princess was chained as a sacrifice to a sea monster because her mother had bragged about her beauty. Then down into the Old City to buy jewellery before picking up Anna's rucksack and taking a taxi to the airport. Anna was interrogated while I stood there helpless and wished for a more dignified parting. And then it was upon us; the time to say goodbye. We kissed passionately and hugged. I turned to go then grabbed her again. Neither of us cried. Then I left the airport walking backwards looking at her, and opened her note in the bus queue even though I'd promised to wait until I was going to sleep. I read it and cried in front of everyone, then cried again when I read it on the bus:

Keep flying, keep going, will be thinking of you always. Take care, be happy, laugh and smile and you'll be a winner. You must be anyway — you survived three and a half months of me! We've got brilliant memories of Afiq, Jerusalem and everywhere else so don't forget them and in three years' time we'll travel far away and make many more memories. I think I'll miss you more than you realise, so please don't forget to keep in touch. Remember me. Good luck in everything. Love you forever — Anna xxx

I turned it over and looked at the picture; our Sea of Galilee. And the floodgates opened once more. I got off the bus early, walked for an hour feeling so alone; no Anna, not even Helen or Rob. Then back to the hostel, I talked to nobody, drank vodka, wrote to my girl, wrote that when I was back in London arranging things I'd dreamt about meeting a girl in Israel, a girl I could fall in love with and travel the world with. And what happened? I fell in love with the only girl out of six that had to go back to England. I wrote for an hour non-stop, put my head on the pillow and cried myself to sleep.

Colleagues welcome Tony back to work whilst sorting files and personal alarms, slugging down coffee before heading off to wings and workshops. Tony's been with his sister, driving through Holland and France, up to Venice for a few days then back to County Durham. I didn't think about Paul standing beside us, asked Tony if he regularly went on holiday with his sister, said it was something I'd love to do, just time alone, rediscovering each other, finding out about one of the people you should know best but somehow don't. We don't see enough of each other, my sister and I, haven't done since we were children. And we didn't appreciate each other's company back then. Tony sees plenty of his sister. They live close by. Then I notice Paul looking down at the floor, realise what an idiot I've been. His sister died of cancer two years ago. Younger than Anna, she left a grief stricken husband and a bewildered small child behind. He doesn't agree with the medical approach to cancer, says he's researched it fully. Wished he'd started earlier because he was too late to save his sister's life. He believes in diet, in vitamins and supplements. He believes in almond kernels. I don't apologise to him though because he's not looking my way. I simply walk off as fast as I can, pick my files up and get out the room.

I'm working in the Dangerous and Severe Personality Disorder Unit, reading quotes on the wall, waiting for the men to arrive. Wise men speak because they have something to say. Fools speak because they have to say something. And then the men enter and one of them gives me his story entitled The Explosion of Krakatoa. After half an hour on that I'm sat with someone else, a man confused about Sikhism. He's got some information from Encyclopaedia Britannica but it talks about miracles and prophecies and he states they aren't allowed in Sikhism. Also, how can one Guru be revered but then his tenth book discredited? His Dad hadn't told him this. According to the paper in front of him Guru Gobind Singh was hounded out, took part in extortion, also illegal in Sikhism, and was then killed in 1708. The student's not angry. He's just confused. He's obsessive compulsive, focused on perfection, order and control. He doesn't know what to think now.

Donations over the last fortnight are as follows:

Banana cake baked by Annette

Coffee and walnut cake baked by my sister

A bottle of whisky from Anna's Dad

Three bottles of homebrew wine (year and contents unknown), one large cabbage, a big bag of leeks, a bag of salad leaves, spinach, parsley, a bag of apples, a home baked apple cake, a box of homemade fairy cakes, six eggs, a tub of fruit salad and a gooseberry crumble, all from Lin.

Isla wants her Mammy to put her to bed and read stories, not me. She repeats it over and over again.

"Mama...Mama"

I help her out her clothes.

"Mama...Mama"

Eventually she lets me help with pyjamas too. And I read her a book in bed before she quickly falls asleep, hair fanned out over pillow, little fist clenching rabbit. When Anna finishes with Joe she shows me what she's planted while I've been at work; salad leaves, radishes, carrots, early and late purple sprouting broccoli, baby and normal turnips, beetroot, peas, runner beans, fennel, basil, sweet peas and purple sprouts, whatever they are. She's also unblocked the drains, done the washing and taken Joe to the doctors after school. She goes and puts her wig on, just for half an hour. But her eyes are tired so she takes her contact lenses out as well. Perhaps the glasses don't help but it looks so obviously like a wig, it really does. She sees me staring, looks uncomfortable, gives a rueful smile.

"It needs to settle down. It's already a bit better than it was"

"Come here," I say.

She walks over. I smooth the sides down, lean back and look again, tell her she looks like Maureen Lipman's younger sister. She laughs, but not because she thinks my comment funny. Then gently, I put it behind her head in a ponytail, try a few different styles. It feels intimate doing this, as if I'm playing with a real part of her.

"It looks better already"

"Does it?"

"Yeah. And it will look even better when your real hair's gone"

She doesn't look too sure. I start to regret my insensitive joke.

"Honest, it does. It just takes few minutes to get used to it, that's all"

The bus dropped me off in the middle of the Negev Desert. I looked around, saw nothing but dry sand, dust in the distance as the bus shimmered away in the heat towards mirage mountains. The road to the left seemed to lead nowhere. I emptied a few sunflower seeds into my palm, munched them and rolled a cigarette. Then I heaved the rucksack on my back, blew out smoke and tramped down the middle of the road, hoping to God there'd be work because I'd spent the last of my money on bus ticket, tobacco and seeds.

Within a kilometre of walking I'd been picked up and given a lift the remaining three kilometres. And there, in the middle of the baking hot desert, I arrived at Ein Yahav, a broad scattering of low slung buildings. I walked up to a house pointed out to me, was told to "come back tomorrow," then taken to house 114 and left to introduce myself to a man from South Africa, a man from Oxford and a Maori from New Zealand. They told me moshavs were not friendly kibbutzim. Everyone was forced to work much harder. And if you were deemed not good enough you were sacked on the spot. The pub was like the Wild West. Fights broke out every night. Chairs over heads. People being punched through windows. Every one of the two hundred Thai men present had been banned from there because they reacted with swift violence whenever antagonised by drunken Englishmen and others. And although it was highly unlikely they'd all reacted in such a manner the Israelis couldn't tell them apart so banned them all. They were there to send money back to their families, saving their main priority. And every time they had one of their special meals a few dogs and cats went missing. I spent the night on a hard floor, woke up freezing and aching, went to find the woman who gave jobs out. But after not finding her at the office or at her house I did as I was advised the previous night and started banging on doors. After an hour I was disillusioned with rejections, annoyed with growling dogs and ready to pack it all in. But I sat down and read Anna's note instead.

Keep flying, keep going.....and you'll be a winner

At two p.m., the 51st house I'd banged on, I found a farmer

called Eilan who needed to hire someone. He took me to the smallest and shabbiest house ever, introduced me to Gary from South Africa and Ray from Ireland, who I had to share a room with. I sat up talking with them, relieved at another new start, wrote a few lines to Anna. Then went to bed early, ready to start work in the morning. Seven days a week, twelve hours a day.

I leave Anna with a kiss and drive to work. She's taking Isla to playgroup for the last time. Making dinner for them both before leaving Isla with Claire and getting the bus to North Tyneside General for her first session of chemotherapy. I walk past lots of prison officers still sat in cars, wonder what's going on. By the time I get to the gate there's a large cluster of them hanging around. After making my way through the security procedures and the plethora of locked gates, I arrive in the staffroom and see another staff notice has been changed. 'UCU meeting required to elect rep' has now become 'UCU meeting required to electrocute rep.' The morning's classes are delayed because the governor has called a meeting. An officer says it's about prisons getting privatised, what the government calls restructuring. I hang around with my colleagues but my heart and head remain back at the coast. And I dive out the way of people's sneezes as if they were germ warfare attacks.

I look at her differently. Study her face, her hair. Look for changes, though I'm not sure I can see any yet. She shows me the central line sticking out of her, says she's sore on both sides now. Louise and Anna's Mum leave, looking guilty for doing so but knowing there's nothing else they can do, not for now.

Anna doesn't try her wig on tonight. She sits on the couch and reads a magazine until ten p.m. because she can take steroids then to combat nausea. She's tired physically but mentally wide awake. Says she could stay on the couch the whole of the next six weeks.

I wake up with Isla climbing over me, getting into the middle of us. Anna says she was awake anyway, can't actually remember getting any sleep. I warn Isla three times to be careful. There isn't any side it's okay to press down on now. I kiss Anna good morning, wonder if her face is thinner, quickly scan her hair, hope she doesn't notice. Anti-nausea tablets come up with her mug of tea and I also wonder if you're waiting to feel sick, waiting for what energy you do have to be syringed out of you, does the thought of it have any impact? Will it make it more likely to happen? And will it happen quicker?

I wash and condition her hair as she sits in the bath like one of our children. Explain to Joe and Isla they'll have to wait for their porridge, if Anna could wash her own hair she would. Anna apologises for the tenth time, stretches out for her cup of tea, takes a sip and pulls a face. Chemotherapy messes around with your taste buds, she says. Like pregnancy.

Anna stays inside and goes back to bed. I take the kids with Helen and Jimmy, Arthur and Eleanor. We pick Billy up on the way, head down the beach for a couple of hours, dig holes that fill with water, put a catfish and three crabs in. Climb sand dunes and throw the ball for Caffrey. Then back home we go, girls on shoulders, for cottage pie that Building Granny brings, cooked with Lin's spinach, who arrives later with homemade apple and gooseberry crumble and minestrone soup. Anna never did go back to bed. She was outside in the back garden when we came home, always was a sun worshipper. She looks fantastic, like nothing has happened. After dinner she takes the kids to Billy's pirate party, leaves me at home for two hours so I can transfer scribbling from paper to computer. It's like the old days. But when she comes home she sticks her tongue out and it smells foul, is coated white all over.

I woke at six every morning, worked in the fields all day. Picked peppers, tomatoes, onions, pumpkins and aubergines. I planted melons and made box after box after box from flat-packed cardboard. Saw very little of anyone but Gary and Ray. House 114 would have been much better fun but I would have spent my money on alcohol if I'd stayed there. Instead, I managed to save three out of five shekels every day. After work we ate only bread and cheese, sometimes a little fruit, fot there was no such thing as free food. Then the other two went inside and had a cold shower - our house had no hot water and no heaters, not even a stove to heat water up on. I sat outside on an ancient armchair that crawled with insects, smoked cigarettes, listened to cockerels. Then I'd go into our tiny dump and chat. We did have fun but I had to listen to Gary talk politics, insult Britain and America, the 'kafirs' back home. And Ray was not the most cheerful. He'd come to Israel to travel, not work. But he'd brought four hundred Irish pounds and couldn't get anyone to change them. When we were too tired to talk or argue we went back to our bedrooms, freezing because the desert nights came in sharp. Ray went to sleep and I laid on my wooden door on metal tables masquerading as a bed and wrote to Anna. And then I fell asleep too. And eventually morning came, with more of the same. And it was back to dry fields, with nothing for scenery but a vast horizon of sandy soil that stretched as far as the eye could see. I crouched and picked, crouched and picked, all day long under a burning sun until my back threatened to snap, occasionally looking up and focusing on the far distance where, if I concentrated hard, the faint outline of mountains could just about be made out.

PART VI

Colleagues ask how the weekend was. I tell them it was fine and there's a pause while they try and work out if I'm telling the truth or avoiding it. Then they ask how Anna is, because they feel they should, and because they care. I photocopy poetry by Roger McGough, Sylvia Plath and Tupac Shakur, requested by students last week when they didn't take to the poems I brought in. I couldn't find Patrick Neate, chuck Wilfred Owen and Brian Patten in instead.

And then I'm in the class. And I'm the teacher. I'm the one stood in front, the one teaching skills to those that need them. The one they should be grateful to, because not many people want to work inside a prison and many think they shouldn't have access to education anyway, that they should be locked up with the key thrown away, either that or electrocuted. But I've realised in the last year I can learn just as much from my students as they can from me, more in fact. One of my students is the same age as me but has been in prison for twenty years. He's changed from someone who would resort to violence at the slightest trigger to someone who can quote the Bible, the Koran, has completed a degree in psychology. But when it comes to mobile phones and the internet, he's amazed such things exist, has never used them, never had access to them. Just read about them in the newspapers, seen them on telly. He's got a daughter who's grown from a baby into a toddler, into a child and then a teenager. She's now a young adult and she's only seen her Daddy on a few occasions and only then for an hour in prison visiting time. My student says he's changed, has had plenty of time to do so, understands how he used violence to control others, to hide his own insecurities and perceived inabilities. I believe him but it seems many don't, for he still doesn't know when his release date will be.

Another student comes from a gypsy family, travelled as a young man through India and Afghanistan helping make deals with drug barons and warlords. He tells about life in the Hindu Kush, about villages where entire profits come from fixing old guns, of young children with fingers missing because they were the ones that had to test them first. Of old women boiling marijuana in huge vats, scraping resin off the top with planks of wood. And many of my students are politically aware, much more than I am. They watch the news, Question Time and Panorama religiously. They often ask if I've watched such and such a programme, if I have any views on the subject. I usually answer with a shrug, say I don't watch TV. I don't tell them I'm too busy living my life but I reckon they can guess. And I presume we can both see the irony of it all; that they, who are locked up behind concrete walls and razor wire, are infatuated with what's happening out there in the big wide world. While I, free as I am, often don't have time or inclination.

I drive home through spring rain, find Joe, Isla and Anna cuddling up, eating peanuts and watching telly. Anna looks fantastic. She walked Joe and Isla to school and child-minder this morning, came back to find a vegetable lasagne on the doorstep, had fish fingers, courgette and mashed potato for breakfast then spent the day resting. We put the kids to bed, eat hotdogs, tidy up and go to bed early ourselves. I watch her get undressed, one side of her chest completely flat now, the cut from one side to the other healing nicely. The other side a beautiful breast, isolated on its own. But this second breast has not been completely left alone. There's gauze where the central line was inserted into the top of it, a tube sticking out further below that swings as she stoops to take off knickers. She gets into bed, starts to read The Other Hand. I fall asleep with unused pen and paper.

Nine days and nights without alcohol or tobacco. It's nothing for some people, mountains and milestones for others. Me, I'm quietly pleased with myself when I wake up. The energy is back in my legs. My head is clearer. It's not difficult. It's just taking a decision and having the will to stick with it for the first couple of days in order to establish a new pattern. Then taking it day by day, hour by hour if necessary. I crunch my almond kernels. Anna won't have them so I've decided to eat them instead, am crunching a relatively safe three a day. Then I walk Caffrey, leave Anna feeling sick, slumped in bed with Isla and a book about shapes.

They don't know how important they are. How could they? I've never told them. Sometimes I walk into the staffroom and a smirk instantly comes across my face. Andy's constant quips, his side-kick Bill. Tony, Dave, the other Andy. Immediacy and wit. Clever or childish but always funny. Rambling tales from Moira. Kim singing while everyone else arrives and scurries round. Sometimes I can't stop laughing at work. There isn't a chance to pause. They come too fast, one after the other, from all directions, and it's difficult to even eat on such occasions. And then there's the understanding glances, the hand on the shoulder, the cuddles, just a look from Kathleen, Margaret, Jean, Izzy, Lynne, Louise and others. And the boss that has constant staffing issues, who is being pulled in different directions but always allows time off without question.

My plan was to work non-stop for four months. Do as much overtime as I possibly could then travel around Egypt before heading off to Greece for work in tourist resorts. But moshav work was tough, Eilan the boss gruff and unthankful, despite the fact we all worked extremely hard for such little reward. Three Thai men came to work with us but they didn't fit the stereotype I'd been given. They spoke no English but were very friendly. And they worked twice as fast as we could. Gary meanwhile, acquired a new girlfriend from Dover called Claire, spent time with her. Left me and Ray to our miserable selves most of the time. I wrote to Anna every night, sent my letter after five or six

170

days. I sent it to her Mum's house, knowing it would have to be sent on from there. Wondered how long it would be before she sent one back. Realised it would take a week for it to arrive with me, presuming both letters made their way through the postal systems without hindrance. I drew dark pictures, wrote my first poetry. Went two months without shaving. Didn't wash for four or five days at a time, didn't brush teeth too much either. Didn't see the point. Eilan started to get annoyed with me, said I wasn't picking enough for him to make a profit. He made me work alone in the packing sheds. I worked harder, couldn't afford to get sacked. Kept going until I'd completed a fourteen hour shift, then went and blasted the overtime at the pub. For the first time I met loads of other people, got drunk, danced and forgot about feeling miserable. The next day I checked for post as usual, and as usual still didn't have any. I wondered if Anna would forget about me and start seeing someone else. Imagined all the lads flocking round student nurses. I flicked my cigarette stub into the sandy dirt and tried to imagine where Anna was right then, what she was doing while I was sat in that insect infected armchair. And then I lit another cigarette and hoped she was sat alone and miserable, just like me.

"If you could be any animal in the world, what would it be?"

"Am I allowed to pick birds?"

"Yeah course. Whatever"

"An eagle"

My student looks disappointed.

"People always pick that"

"Wouldn't you like to fly?" I ask him. "Jump off a mountain and soar? And you'd want to be top of the food chain surely?"

"I'd be a whale," he says, dismissing a suggestion of crocodile from across the room with a wave of the hand.

"You don't want to soar?"

"No man. I'd be a whale. Whales have got it sorted, have got everything an animal needs. They don't feel stress because they have food all around them whenever they need it. They don't have anything that hunts them, as long as they stay away from man. They spend all their time with family and friends, have nothing to do but eat and relax with those they love, those that are close to them. And then, every six months or something, they go on a journey together, migrate to the other side of the world. That's what life should be like"

The rest of the class go quiet for a second, then turn into nodding dogs.

I drive home through pouring rain to find Isla asleep, Anna in bed with Joe reading Feefo, Jinks and Tuppeny. I leave them to it, come back downstairs, find Isla's new school cardigan, red with a white badge, still in cellophane. I imagine her in it tomorrow, just turned three, jumping up and down in excitement as she goes to school, nervous too perhaps. It melts me, thinking of her in that uniform, wondering where the last three years have gone, how quickly my beautiful little girl is growing up. I can remember my

Mam taking photographs of me in my school uniform, my cub scout uniform. I didn't see the point at the time, found it an intrusion to have to stay still, even for a minute. We go to bed talking about Isla's first day tomorrow, wondering how she'll be. Anna puts her hand to her head, says it feels weird, tingling. She pulls at her hair, then looks at her fingers, but there's nothing there. Not yet.

Isla comes to our bedroom at half five, stands just inside the doorway.

"It's too early Isla. Go back to bed please"

She doesn't move.

"Go back to bed Isla. It's too early"

The sides of her mouth turn down and she goes back out. I hear her climb into bed, cry "Mammy" a few times. And then it goes quiet.

She comes in again just after six, smiles joyfully when I beckon her to climb in. Cuddles up to both of us, puts her arm around us in turn. Strokes our faces.

"Where are you going today?" asks Anna.

Her eyes roll around, searching.

"Don't know"

"School"

Isla beams, excitement in her eyes. But then, after ten seconds or so, she looks doubtful, cries for Mammy again, this time throws her arms around her. We make coffee and warm milk as a distraction. It works for a few seconds but then she gets back into bed and says she feels sick. And although breakfast goes down no bother, when she walks into the kitchen, uniform on and hair platted, she's starting to have doubts once more.

"I feel sick"

"Do you?"

"Yeah"

"Whereabouts do you feel sick?"

"Everywhere except my hands and my eyeballs"

"Oh right"

Then she spots me making my breakfast.

"What have you got?"

I don't need to answer. She sees the tub.

"But yoghurt makes me better"

"Does it?"

And she swaggers to the table. Boasting to Joe she's having yoghurt for breakfast and he's not.

Anna goes to hospital for a check up but makes sure she's back to pick Isla up. Neither of us want to miss her coming out after her first morning at school. She walks out calmly, school bag swinging gently, increasing smile. Then she's right in front of us, so cute and little in her uniform, showing all her teeth inside a beautiful smile. Jumping up and down with uncontainable energy. By the time we've got home though, Anna and I are arguing. Not major arguments. Just tired disagreements. Isla doesn't eat much dinner, puts her head in it twice, isn't allowed pudding and starts to cry. Anna and I argue over how to deal with it. She closes her eyes and refuses to talk to me. I go into the kitchen and crunch apricot kernels.

Anna's getting ready to collect Joe from school. Isla wants to go with her, is grabbing hold of her leg. Anna bends down to get her trainers, notices something. Freezes.

"What's that?"

She picks it up, straightens herself, holds out her hand. It's a clump of hair. Only small. About eight inches long. Perhaps twenty or so strands woven together. She half smiles but we don't have time to talk. She's got to get Joe, and Isla will be with her, chattering on obliviously. Then she'll have parents and friends to talk to in the sunshine as the children run and climb. And she won't be ready to talk about it with anyone else yet.

After weeks of checking the post daily and finding nothing each time, I continued more out of routine than expectation. But when the woman produced an envelope and placed it in my hands it was as if she'd put something in my gut at the same time. I slid it into my back pocket for safekeeping and rushed off to work, savouring it for later, or so I hoped. We sat on the trailer, hung legs over the side, smoked cigarettes as the tractor pulled out into fields. I watched one of the Thai lads fire a homemade catapult at birds and cats as we bumped along, put my hand onto my back pocket, felt the envelope that stuck out and wondered what lay within. The tractor stopped outside the shelter for what I presumed was just another morning of making flat pack boxes. Eilan waited outside but you couldn't tell he had important news by his face or stance. It was simply business as usual for an emotionless farmer who invested in vegetables and didn't give two hoots about people. This business of his had natural peaks and troughs. And we were just about to enter the latter. He let us go inside the shelter first. Then told us there was only one week left of work. After that there was nothing.

I waited until he'd walked back out the shelter and put one of his prized export tomatoes in my mouth. Its juice and seed dribbled down my chin. I wiped myself clean, checked over my shoulder, saw Eilan still outside and stuffed another one in, then another and another. And another. I took the envelope out my pocket, clutched it tight, walked out into dry fields. Didn't know whether to laugh or cry. Eilan wandered off, more important things than people to worry about. I let the others pick and opened my letter. Followed her emotions and thoughts as, like me, she'd written something most days until receiving a letter from me and having an address to send back to. She was lonely at first, very lonely. But as the weeks passed her words became lighter. She'd made good friends and had set about spending her bursary. But still, for five days per week her body was in a classroom without its heart. This was the early stages of Project 2000. The course was more academic than she expected and although she'd attained nine GCSE's she struggled. Working with people would have helped, on wards with those that needed a hand. But she was too busy trying to get her wandering mind around essays and competencies. She knew she had to give nursing a go because it was all she'd ever wanted to do, and there was no money to do anything else anyway. And she desperately hoped we had a future together but was aware that fate had driven us apart and was afraid we would never see each other again. At the bottom of the letter was her address so

I could write directly to her; The Royal Victoria Infirmary, Newcastle upon Tyne. I glanced around, put the letter into my pocket and began to pick, very slowly. Her words were not enough. I needed to know more. What was her work like? What were her friends like? What was a normal day for her? What clothes did she wear? Was she wearing the earring from Jerusalem? The pair she'd made at the market then separated so we could have one each? I had mine in, had never taken it out. I took the letter out and read it again. But this time checked for hidden meanings, became more worried about how it went from depression through to contentment, or at least acceptance. I feared this would lead her to mentally turn away from me, thus creating space for others to fill. After work I wrote back and insisted she tell me immediately if she met someone else. I didn't want to guess from letters, read between lines, sow seeds of doubt that sprouted from ambiguous words. I knew she wouldn't want to hurt my feelings. But I dreaded turning up in Newcastle and seeing in her eyes she wasn't pleased to see me because it put her in an awkward position. And then I called my Mam, got her to contact a florist. Had three red roses sent for Valentine's Day with the message, "from three thousand miles away with love xxx"

We're tidying in the kitchen when Radio 4 tells us 40% of Britain could be infected by Mexican swine flu within the next couple of weeks.

"I know it's silly," says Anna. "But it does make me worried, with my immune system about to be shot to pieces"

Three more people have been found infected in the country. That brings the number up to four so far. Straight after Mexican swine flu comes a story about Barrack Obama. Its one hundred days since he took office. The radio presenter talks about how Obama's been on the road all this time, how he's been trying to turn things round. It must be one hundred days since Anna was diagnosed with cancer. She carries on filling the dishwasher, seemingly oblivious. I decide it's not appropriate to wish her happy anniversary. The presenter completes with a fitting pay off for both the US president and my girl:

"One thing's for sure; he may have come a long way in such a short time but he's still got a long long road to travel"

I'm reading 'If Mum and Me were Mermaids' to Isla in bed. Joe's tucked in next to her, the two of them sandwiched between myself and Anna, Caffrey at our feet. I explain about oysters, point out pearls.

"Yeah I know," says Joe. "Some people say they're mermaids' tears that have been frozen"

I make porridge, listen to Radio 4 tell me eighteen cases of swine flu have now been confirmed in Britain. We eat breakfast, watch two jackdaws flap down into the garden. One lands on the birdhouse, keeps watch, its head jerking sideways to some invisible beat. The other comes down onto grass, struts towards bread that Anna put out. Its head betrays it, twitches sideways nervously, large grey beak thrusting out at would-be rivals; a curious mixture of swagger and paranoia.

Freda from next door comes round with a parcel. I'm on the Internet reading about Tyneside's first swine flu victim. The parcel's addressed to her but has come from a garden centre. She wonders if we ordered it, put her address because we weren't sure if we'd be home or not. I shake my head, tell her it must be for her. Perhaps it's a nice plant sent from someone in her family? It can't be she says. Her family are all in Canada. Either that or on holiday in Mexico. I edge back, my mind forging connections, danger routes to Anna. Half an hour later Anna comes back from the library, says Lin works with the only person in Tyneside confirmed as having swine flu. I tell her about Freda's family on holiday in Mexico. She sighs heavily, goes for a lie down. I take the kids to the new playground with Helen, Jimmy, Arthur and Eleanor. But when we come back she's sat out the back in the sunshine again, says she never went upstairs. I notice but don't say anything. She waits until the kids are happily playing on the grass, puts her hand through her hair and tells me. It's lost its shine, is looking coarse and aged. And it's not just shine either. It's lost its bounce too, is flat to her head. It's lifeless. Dying.

We drive through Whitley Bay in the sunshine. Past bank holiday families walking dogs, eating fish and chips and ice cream. Teenagers showing off bodies, getting tans started for summer. Older people resting on railings. All is quiet inside the car except an old ska CD, playing softly. Anna gazes out the window at everyone lapping up the sun's rays, then brings her head forward and stares aimlessly out the front windscreen. I keep glancing across but she doesn't respond. Her eyes look empty but I know her mind has plenty to occupy it. It's one of those moments when she's lost in a future world of suffering, of her children's fragile mental states, perhaps her own death. But then I notice her finger tapping gently to "Let's do Rocksteady" and I wonder if she's coming back out from wherever she is. But no; she turns her head to look at me and her eyes are a mixture of apprehension and resignation. And then more staring out the window, except this time her finger's continued tapping and is starting to enjoy itself a little bit more. Then her body starts to move too, and before ten seconds is out she's dancing. She turns around and smiles at the children, gets them dancing too. And we drive up past the Spanish City dome with the whole car dancing and smiling along. We have a happy feast in Richard and Louise's garden to celebrate Building Granny's birthday. We watch Richard jump up and down with a barbecue fork, trying to spear a seagull that's shitting on his new conservatory. We talk to children that run and chatter around us, talk about the same children when they play further away from us.

And we talk about children not yet born.

And chemotherapy.

By the time our last day of work came I hadn't washed properly for twelve days, hadn't seen the point. But a new adventure was about to begin, for the three of us had decided to spend a few weeks in Egypt. Except the night before we were due to leave Gary found out his South African passport meant he was banned from visiting Egypt. South Africa and Israel had collaborated on military training, on weapons development and weapons production for years, and now he was going to pay his small price for it. We went to see Eilan to get our money, to check if we could leave our belongings in the house. He said we could, that we should come back in a few weeks, there might be some work on. Ray and I got two bottles of vodka and proceeded to get drunk. Gary hated alcohol, was teetotal, got more irritated the drunker we got. And by the end of the night he was fuming because his girlfriend Claire helped us finish the vodka and decided she would travel to Egypt with us.

Life is vicious and indiscriminate. It swipes away lives at random, crushes families or pulls them apart, infects and sickens. Sometimes, music feels like all we have. It helps us drive to work when our minds are a million miles away. Its drum establishes rapport with our heartbeat, echoes wild frustrations and anger. Guitars that can turn over tanks, or simply make us want to dance. Because life can be joyous too, thank God. And friends often gather round in times of difficulty. Music helps us celebrate, lose our inhibitions, our fears, our virginity. It trivialises, puts smiles on faces, allows for reflection and introspection. I'm on my way back from seeing Frankie and the Heartstrings play their second ever gig, at the Tyne pub on Newcastle's quayside. I've had a few beers and I'm wondering if music and literature have something in common, if fashion and connection overpower and accelerate past talent. I'm wondering if the Heartstrings and myself will be left behind by those from the right location, with the accident of better timing. By those that look for bandwagons to jump on as soon as they notice them moving. On the metro seat opposite, some drunken lad has his hands on a girl's knees. He leans forwards and asks for a kiss but she ignores him, keeps on talking. Then he grabs the back of her head, pushes her forwards towards him and plants his mouth on hers. She pulls away, tells him to stop but keeps her legs out front and on top of his. I realise they've just met tonight. He asks where she lives, what she does for a job. Then they get off and I watch them walk down the platform together, side by side but not holding hands. And I wonder how their night will end...

This younger lad gets on through the same doors, doesn't come towards the seats, turns round as the doors slide shut, faces them, back to everyone else as the metro moves away. I stare at the back of his head, am sure I know him but can't place where from. He turns around, looks at me briefly but shows no sign of recognition on his face. And then I remember. A year and a half ago I was asked to spend the day with a twelve year old who was having problems. His father wasn't present the majority of the time, was violent when he was. My boss thought he would benefit from some male supervision and guidance before I went back to the homeless hostel being refurbished. The Family Intervention Team didn't have any male workers. I turned up at school with Rachel, his key-worker. We were met at the front door by the Education Social Worker and the Head of Year. They explained he was only allowed in school for two hours in the morning, that this was a cautious step in the right direction as he'd been completely suspended for a number of months. We walked into his classroom. He was on top of the wardrobe, facing the windows, the only one there. Ignoring all attempts to rationalise. He was up there because he didn't want to leave at the end of his two hours. He wanted to stay and do more work. An hour later he was running to the Baltic Art Museum, Rachel and I trying to keep up. Another hour later, Rachel asked him if he wanted to meet up with me again. He said he did, asked if I played football. I said I loved playing football, would love to meet up with him again too. But I hesitated, said it would be up to my boss, not me. I chatted about it with Rachel after we dropped him off home. Realised the homeless hostel would be re-opening in three months and I'd be working there full time with new management, new structures and policies. The next day I told my boss I wouldn't see the lad again. I wouldn't work with him for three months, have him disclose personal issues and dreams, develop a relationship with him and then dump him. He glances around the metro once more, still shows no sign of recognition, exudes boredom more than anything else. Then he gets off with that teenage swagger, doesn't look back. And I think, even if he had recognised me, he'd only have seen another worker, yet another worker who'd let him down and left him.

I'm on the computer checking e-mails. I have an interview with Isolationist, a North East arts and culture website that wants to push me as a local writer. Anna comes up and I gently lean my head on her, not realising there's anything different at first. Then I remember my head shouldn't be nestled between two curves. I look up and she stops stroking my hair.

"Prosthesis"

"Excuse me?"

"I've got a new breast. Do you want to see it?"

"Err, yeah. Go on then"

She reaches inside her bra and takes it out. Kneads it in her hand like dough.

"Do you want to have a feel of it?"

My face must be a right picture.

"Well, no not really"

But Anna looks playful.

"Go on," she says, holding it out. "Take it. It feels really nice"

So I hold it in my hand and squash it like a stress ball while she tells me her hair is coming out faster. Then I give her it back and she goes to put her wig on.

She trips over my chair leg, spills carrot and coriander soup over her hand and the floor, swears and runs for cold water. Comes back five minutes later when I've wiped it all up, says she doesn't like it anyway. Then she runs her hand over her head, pulls out hairs. Rolls them into a ball. Rolls them between thumb and forefinger making a wiry scratchy sound. Puts the finished result on the table.

"How come you're allowed to do that?" I ask. "I'm not allowed to put toe-nails there"

"That's different," she tells me.

She walks away, head down. Comes back with more. Places them on the table as well.

"They're appearing all over the house," she says. "I'm moulting.....I'm worse than the dog"

Perhaps it's the wrong chapter. After all, I only chose it ten seconds before going on. Or perhaps it's the wrong audience. Or maybe it's that the audience are captivated and clinging to every word and that's why they don't remember to laugh in the right places. I step off the stage without looking at them, all seventeen of them. Walk the short distance back to my seat. At least I can sit down now and watch the rest without worry. The interval brings compliments that help reinforce confidence. But I can't answer questions about how well sales are going. I've no idea I say. I presume it's doing well amongst people that know me, okay in the north east of England and probably nothing whatsoever everywhere else. I do manage to sell one though, make myself a net profit of three pounds. I think about the three years it took to write as I pocket the money, how it won't even cover half the petrol money to get here and back. Then Jeff comes over, a seasoned performance poet for over ten years. He picks up a copy, reads the cover note, says he'd like to buy one. But it seems wrong to agree when he has a book for sale too.

"Fancy a swap?" I ask.

And so we do. He tells me he came to the Bridge Hotel twenty, thirty years ago. It was the meeting place for every left leaning political group in Newcastle. They all had a room each, never mingled. Viewed each other as the enemy as much as they did the right. Then he asks how sales are going.

"I've no idea," I say. "I don't think I'm rich yet"

"Aye; films is where it's at." He jabs a finger at my book. "You won't make any money out of this"

I give my excuses, say I need to use the toilet before the readings resume.

"That's where the socialist workers party used to meet," says Jeff.

She rolls her hand over her hair, collects a dozen or more strands.

"I'm getting bald patches"

"No you're not," I say. "It's getting thinner but you're hardly bald yet"

But she shows me either side of her parting and she's right.

"I want you to cut it off tonight," she says. "I want to take control of it, not just let it happen. Okay?"

I nod my head and look away.

It connects the Mediterranean to the Red Sea, was cut out from earth using forced labour, opened in 1869 and allowed transportation between Europe and Asia without the need for navigation around Africa. Over 1.5 million people from numerous countries were employed by the Suez Canal Company, with thousands dying in the ten years it took to complete. The place was almost deserted when we were there though. Just a broad expanse of deepening blue sky, a gentle tide that rippled from one sea to another. Occasional grey tankers that moved slowly through like giant metal whales. On the far side; undulating sand banks decorated with palm trees, the start of the Sinai desert we'd travelled through for the last five hours. I ate a chewy burger that tasted of camel worked to death. Listened to a Colombian guy play a pink guitar, talk about the Oxford Hotel, how it was the cheapest place to stay in Cairo. He was with two other guys, all with long hair and homemade jewellery, one from Israel and the other an Indian with a flute. They'd had a joint in Tel Aviv before boarding the bus and had become overtly paranoid at the border crossing but were now beginning to chill out again. The Oxford Hotel contained plenty of cannabis they said, was the centre of the black market trade. We were ushered back on the bus and I took my seat next to Claire. Ray, behind us, had already moaned a great deal. Wished he was back in a pub in Ireland, could watch his favourite telly programmes. Claire talked about Buddhist retreats in India, of books and meditation. She smoked cannabis and was up for an adventure. She and I were on the same wavelength, Ray an accepted but quiet and grumbling companion. Gary seethed and simmered. But he was out of sight and out of mind back at the moshav.

The door needs a kick to help it open. Flakes of blue paint drop to the floor as the door bounces off the wall behind and then comes back again, reluctant to reveal what lies inside. But in we go, to a dark and dusty corridor. Squares of light coming in from a side office, highlighting a large mahogany clocking in machine.

Dawn looks back and smiles.

"Come up here," she says.

We go carefully up dirty stairs, turn right onto the shop floor.

"This is the third time I've been in," she says. "It's changing all the time. That corrugated roof pane has fallen down"

Sunshine beams down through the gap. Bits of ceiling and wall collapsed.

"Time moves on. The pigeons have moved in. Everything changes"

This shop fitters and joinery specialists covers three floors, once employed over a hundred men, first started operating in 1918. In three months the building, situated in the centre of Sunderland, will be smashed to pieces, torn down by men in hard hats with machines. There's been no one working here in over three years, since the owner went bankrupt. Dawn's been given the keys to make art with anything left behind. With anything she can carry. First she'll make her own art, then she'll have workshops with the community, creating what they want to see in its place, whilst at the same time, two or three streets away, everything that's left, and all it stood for, will be destroyed. I'm excited, a child with a new playground, unable to speak, open mouthed in wonder. Grateful for a day like this when the night promises gut-wrenching emotion and a harsh reality much closer to home. We walk forwards in silence, our eyes adjusting to what little light windows covered in dirt and mesh allow inside. Clamps hold together wood formed into cabinets for the latest shop to fit. Strange shaped tools set down in mid use at the day's end lie coated in dust. They all thought they were coming back to work the next day. Then out through the fire exit we go, with views of school fields, sounds of excited children. Up rotting wooden steps, over a decomposing pigeon and cider bottle shards. Into the owner's penthouse apartment, all columns and curves. Up wide stairs, portholes either side that look out to sea. Across the spacious main room, light-fittings smashed on the floor, electric cables hanging from holes in the ceiling. Trapped inside these elegant half moon walls lie the remnants of what was once a great life, day to day conveniences that money, once taken for granted, bought in droves. All of it dumped in piles and boxes, gathering dust for no one. We walk about with quiet footsteps, as if sudden noise might stir trapped spirits, tumble pans and crockery stacked precariously. A snapped CD and an open bag of sugar. Cups with mouldy tea bags inside, hardened green stains cracked like marble. Bottles of single malt, Moet and Chandon, wine and vodka, all empty. Next to crumpled brown take-away bags and pizza boxes with crusted veins of cheese. And on the right; a flattened pile of birthday cards. Only one still standing, dedicated to 'my son.'

Into the kitchen. Dying plants on the windowsill. Only the top cupboards remain but the doors have disappeared, leave their contents on display like a heartless museum of mockery. Coffee pots, spaghetti, extra virgin olive oil, apple chutney with west country cider, baby beetroot and hoi sin sauce, balsamic vinegar and milk the colour of urine. Touching things seems wrong but I can't help myself. I'm a voyeur with the guilt of a burglar. Dawn leaves. She's seen this before. I walk over to the calendar on the wall, still stuck on June 2007. On the 15th it says 'Father's Day, on the 16th 'Sold Watch £650' and on the 17th 'Phone Bill £370.' I take the calendar off the wall, flip back to May, a picture of Durham Cathedral. On the 14th it says 'MAM DIED', the only writing in capital letters. I put it back, decide I've seen enough, turn round to bottles still full of anti-depressants and antibiotics.

Then back towards the front door I go, snooker room on my left, beautiful full size table in perfect condition. After this a child's bedroom, clothes flung on floor, cupboard doors open. In the first: bright coloured plastic hangers, a giant Incredible Hulk hand, two crutches and Christmas wrapping paper. Nothing in the second but the third full of games and Playmobil boxes. For a moment I consider stealing some of these for my son. He would love them. But I can't bring myself to do it, even though the machines will come and smash all this to pieces. I find the bathroom instead. Jacuzzi, bath and toilet all taken off somewhere else. A large walk in shower still intact, big enough for two or three people to fit in. Shampoo, conditioners and shower gel still on shelves. A wrung out flannel that looks sodden but must have dried solid around the pole. Then the main bedroom, with cupboards open, twenty or thirty shirts of many colours, a previous life of rainbow prosperity. Dawn comes in behind. I ask if she's okay. She feels uncomfortable, she says. There's definitely a story here but it's not hers to tell. As we walk out the bedroom she points at something I've missed, scattered on the living room floor. I crouch down and pick a few coloured shreds up, turn them over in my hand, let them scatter to the floor once more. Credit cards. Two or three of them. Cut into tiny glittering pieces.

Emo Phillips stood for half an hour with his arms out wide, stared at the wall. Then he turned around and talked about the oneness of being, about Morocco and visions of countryside in the air. And then he sat on the floor, crossed legs and rolled a joint. Now this may have been the first joint I'd smoked in five long months but I swear there was something else other than cannabis inside it. Someone would say something and everyone would stare for fifteen minutes. Then someone would remember the point and answer, upon which the whole process would start again. And when you focussed on something the image repeatedly flashed in your brain for the next five minutes. Ray and Claire crashed out almost immediately. Or maybe they just needed to get away, were pretending to be asleep. I sat there while Emo Phillips talked to the wall. And then I started to feel paranoid, that he was waiting for us all to fall asleep so he could kill us. I went onto my balcony six floors up, wrote thirty lines to Anna that seemed to take forever and needed ridiculous amounts of concentration. Watched people and cars below. But the paranoia returned in dark shivering waves and I wondered why the person in the room behind had spent the last hour and a half cutting sellotape. And I was scared to walk back in because that person had seen me a couple of hours ago and I was normal back then. But I realised Emo Phillips would come through the door and push me over the balcony. And so I managed to light a Cleopatra cigarette and go back to my own room. Four Germans were in there playing guitar and smoking joints and they looked concerned about me. I kept staring at the wall and forgetting what I was doing. But eventually, after an hour or so, I managed to get my legs into the sleeping bag and collapse into darkness.

The light doesn't shine so brightly through the corrugated plastic roof tiles now I'm back downstairs. My excitement of earlier seems downright inappropriate. I'm more aware of the emptiness, not the clutter. The almost silence. Wind gently rattling through gaps. A flutter of pigeon wings. This place would have been full of noise, full of life, of shouting and laughter, of machinery and careful calculation. There's history here, of many people over many years. And once there was a current with a future imagined. I'm standing in the current now, the deathly stillness of calm before storm, when the settled dust will rise again. Only this time much higher than ever before, as the machines move in and the walls come crashing down. In 1918, when this place first opened, Lawrence of Arabia rode through Damascus in triumph. The Red Baron was shot down in flames and votes were given to women over the age of thirty. Church bells rang as excited boy scouts cycled through town, sounding the all clear on bugles and sirens. And the population of Sunderland rushed out waving flags and shooting off fireworks as one million British soldiers rotted in the ground. Through the Great Depression this place went, and seventy-five per cent unemployment, as it hammered and sawed towards war and bombardment. It survived Hitler and the bombs that rained down, week after week, year after year on Sunderland, the world's biggest shipbuilding town. It survived Thatcher too, as batons cracked heads and the shipyards were sacrificed for Scotland's benefit. And so it continued, providing food on plates and futures of hope and better lives. Until the twenty-first century came along and held out the flat of its palm. And the council refused to budge, refused to allow desperate applications for change of use.

Dawn takes me downstairs into dark offices. I pull out drawers, look through files of jobs already done; jewellers, off-licences, churches, car salesrooms, dentists, pharmacy's, nightclubs. Out to Durham, down to Sheffield, up to Edinburgh. Above them, the in-tray and prospective quotes they didn't get the chance to fulfil. Two primary schools, one for four thousand pounds, another for more than twenty-four thousand. Thirty-six thousand for a company in Washington, two and a half for a shop in Newcastle's Groat Market. Thirty-two thousand for Age Concern. Thirty-five for a Pet and Garden Centre and nine for an insurance company. I wonder if that work could have saved them, or if it went elsewhere because the quotes were higher than average because of desperation for survival. Did the company investigate the proposals and give the quotes knowing it was unlikely they'd be around to undertake the work? Or did the managing director keep the financial problems to himself as long as he could, before calling a meeting and telling everyone they were losing their jobs? I think back to his penthouse apartment, remember those empty bottles of whisky, the full bottles of anti-depressants. I stay still for a moment and listen. Nothing except faint rain trickling and dripping its way through somewhere, finding its path. The occasional tap of something. The creak of something else.

I walk behind the desk, turn over photos of the lads in the pub. Back in the times when they'd have docked off and gone for a few pints together. I look at their faces, their relaxed smiles, wonder if the same lads still meet up, if they've all got work or if some are still signing on. Or if some got work and then lost it again in this recession. On the windowsill above, in front of metal bars and filthy windows; two smurfs, a felt parrot and some reading glasses caked thick in dust. I lift up one of the smurfs because he's facing the wrong way. Dust flicks up, catches sunlight that slides between bars, glitters like fairy dust and settles into ash grey once more. I place the smurf facing the room like his friend then wonder if he preferred to look out the window instead. I sit down in the chair, survey the room in front of me, the hatch on the right where the postman would have arrived, the public too. Next to it; a clock that's come off the wall, fallen onto the counter. Its red pointer still has a tiny spark, is going through the last throes of life, jerks forward a fraction of a second then back again. A limb sticking up, desperate for attention. Stuck on twenty to six. I open the drawers, am greeted by a sickly smell, a 2002 diary. Floppy discs and a ball made of red elastic bands collected from the post. I pick it up, twice the size of a tennis ball, bounce it on the desk and it sounds like it's going to smash right through. Across to the fax machine; its metal drawer stuffed full with faxes that must have come through after the building was finally locked shut. A machine left on, communicating with the outside world, set to automatic menu. I look through the sheets; cars for sale, menu lists from 2007, mince and dumplings, chicken korma, duck wraps, special offers from building suppliers. A questionnaire that will never be filled in. A couple of blank sheets. An error report.

I'd travelled back in time to 2500BC, as long as I continued to look forwards. I lurched up and down, gripped the bobbing neck of my camel, glanced across at a smiling Claire, a frightened looking Ray. Every few minutes our sun scorched guide struck a camel on its behind with a platted rope whip and grinned. I turned to the front and gripped harder as my camel loped down a sandy hill towards small triangles that slowly turned into wonders of the ancient world. Twenty minutes later it was right in front, towering 480 feet above us. The tallest building in the world for 3800 years, built four and a half thousand years ago by four million men using over two million limestone rocks. The Great Pyramid of Giza. Now the colour of the desert sands that slowly shift for hundreds of kilometres, it used to have a smooth outer casing of highly polished white limestone that reflected the desert sun and must have entranced all those lucky enough to have viewed it in its prime. The people of Ancient Egypt believed death on Earth was the start of a journey to the next world. They believed the dark area of the night sky around which the stars appear to revolve was the physical gateway into the heavens. I looked upwards, felt tiny and insignificant in comparison to the colossal size of this ancient building that must have witnessed so much.

Back to Cairo, with its infectious crazed atmosphere, we went down the Nile and climbed the Cairo Tower. We walked through thronged streets, amazed at the sight of so many happy people, the assault of car horns, old men ringing bicycle bells, people leaning out of car windows shouting "welcome" and "tally ho." And then finally, the Oxford Hotel again. And this guy from Bristol who had nothing but the clothes on his body and a didgeridoo. Some German guy gave him a racing bike and off he went, chuffed to bits. Said he was going to cycle all the way to Sudan, his didgeridoo tied on the side with some straggly string. Emo Phillips played some awful music on a flute. Talked about making tunes in the air, how we are all creations apart from God. We left him in his room, found Carlos, Amos and the Indian guy, the three men we'd met on the bus, had a smoke with them instead. Carlos played guitar, the Indian his flute and Amos a plank of wood he took from the bed. Claire and I sang. Amos told us how he'd overdosed on tablets and threatened to kill himself so he could get out the Israeli army. He was classified as medically insane but he was a great drummer. I scratched my insect bites and sang, didn't think about how stupid I was for not having medical insurance, for not having had any jabs and yet eating in the cheapest places Cairo could provide. It was one of the greatest nights ever, one of the reasons I'd started travelling.

The time has come. I have a whisky to top up the strong Belgian beer. Anna has whisky too, a smaller one, while I close the curtains and put both living room lights on. She brings the stool from the kitchen. Sits and watches Gardeners World as if it's just another night. We look at each other and smile. Then I walk up behind, move her slightly so she can turn her head, look in the mirror whenever she wants to. I figure it's better to have that option than to wait until the end and get the shock of your life. And then I take the brush, the idea being to brush as much out as I can first. That way it comes out with the root, leaves less to shave off at the end. I stroke her hair, soft and seemingly in good condition, the recent dead having already departed. But each time I pull the brush through, swirls of brown hair leave her head and curl around the bristles. By the time I've done four brushes they're so tightly packed I have to pull them out with force. I stand with a clump in my hand, ask her what she wants to do with it. Dawn said she could bury it, do something symbolic. Anna says she just wants it put in the bin. So I shove it down as far as it will go and continue brushing, Anna quiet, me finding surprising tenderness in this intimate moment. And then, after about ten minutes, the gaps start to show. White skull shines through and the hair gets thinner and thinner until it becomes so thin I can gather it all up in one hand. Joe appears with a pitter patter down the stairs, says he wants a cuddle. I stand in front of Anna so he can't see. Not when he's supposed to be settling down to sleep. Tell him go back upstairs, someone will be up in ten minutes. And then I brush from underneath, gathering much more. Anna looks in the mirror, smiles nervously, lets her head and neck move with the motion, speaks just once. Tells me it feels nice to have her hair brushed. I try to remember when I last did it but time has erased the memory. And then her hair becomes so thin I have to get scissors. I come back from the kitchen and she's pulled what little hair she has left up into a mad witch look. I brush it back down with my hands, pull it out in isolated strands. Cut it as close to her head as I can with large kitchen scissors. Anna flinches, worried I'll cut her, cause an infection she can't fight off. I reassure, continue until there's just thin wisps on top. And then Joe comes down again, says he's scared, has been looking for dinosaur but can't find him, then looks at his Mammy and laughs, says she "looks funny." I tell him I don't think she does, find dinosaur under the couch, take him back upstairs. Then I come back down again, get the clippers, drop oil onto the blade, push her head down gently and start on the back of her neck. When I'm half way though I turn the clippers off, put them down and walk around in front of her. I bend down so we're on the same level and frown.

She looks at me quizzically. Like she's standing naked in front of a number of people who are expected to honestly comment about her on a live television show. I move forward, kiss her on the head.

"Bloody hell"

"What?"

"You look sexy"

She looks even more quizzical.

"You do, honest"

And it's true. I didn't expect this. I expected her to look terrible, that I'd have to lie. But it suits her, it looks really good. I finish the shaving and she gets up, walks back and forth to the mirror, feeling her head, turning to look from different angles. Her face is plain, just a hint of sparkling bemusement. Like she can't believe this has actually happened. And then she tries her wig on and suddenly it fits so much better, and she walks up and down with that on too, looking in the mirror, flattening it, stroking the fringe this way and that. I grab her close and kiss her, proper kisses this time. And I tell her she looks fantastic.

"Come, come," said the old man, curling his finger and beckoning us inside his small concrete home. We followed him in, left the Karnak Temple in bright sunshine. Stepped into the dark.

"You want hashish?"

A few seconds hesitation. The old man snapped his fingers and shouted something. A girl about five or six years old entered the room then disappeared again at his command. Ten seconds later a woman entered with mint tea, gave us a small cup each.

"Sit," the old man said. "Sit"

He pointed at the only piece of furniture in the room, a small concrete bed with a sheet on. I sat down next to him and Ray did too. But Claire wasn't allowed such luxury. She had to sit on the floor with the woman. The old man lit a joint, took a few drags and passed it to me. I did the same and was prompted to pass to Ray. And then Ray was prompted to pass back to the old man, leaving Claire ignored on the floor. Thirty seconds later two bowls arrived, one filled with cannabis resin, the other with grass.

"Very good hey? You want buy?"

We bought a bit of both, bartered as he brought more young children to smile at us. Then we found our hired bikes and whizzed back towards Luxor, riding the wrong way down a one-way street, weaving in and out of traffic, throwing our heads back and laughing at the blaring horns. The next day we took a horse drawn carriage to the Nile, crossed by ferry and rode donkeys across mountains; just the three of us and our fifteen year old Arab guide. Trotting along cliff edges high above the river, through sugar cane plantations and remote villages. Then down into The Valley of the Kings we went, with blocks of coaches and tourists with I love Egypt hats. Americans who waited for security to disappear then took photographs inside the four thousand year old tombs, even though they were told it could destroy the paintwork and hieroglyphics. When the security guards caught them they asked for five dollars, stuffed it into their pockets. Ray moaned the tombs were boring, wanted to know what was happening in Eastenders. And eventually, we became fed up with being hassled, with always being charged more for our meal than the menu stated. With people wanting money wherever we went. Being told we'd be taken to a beautiful place up the Nile for swimming, then hearing from another traveller that the river was swarming with disease, with insects that burrow into your skin and lay eggs in your bloodstream that hatch. After arguing with the hostel manager about the price for a felucca trip down the Nile we decided to head on. Mohammed had a history of trying to swindle us already. He'd met us at the train station after the 400km journey from Cairo, was the first to mention hot baths. That was the only reason we went to his hostel. But the water never rose as high as luke-warm the four days we were there. And it took a day of reminding to even get a plug.

And so off we went, on the fourteen hour train journey back to Cairo during which Claire dreadlocked my hair, giving the rest of the carriage something to stare at. And then the train further on to Suez but we'd missed the last bus. And so instead of paying a taxi driver seventy pounds we paid a fiver each and hitch-hiked the last section on the back of an open van, one hundred kilometres through desert and mountains in pitch black. We arrived at Dahab and were given a square concrete room with nothing in but three thin mattresses and a candle. But within half an hour we'd got a bag of grass and were lying on the beach, the Sinai mountains where Moses received the Ten Commandments at our backs, wondering why the gorgeous blue water in front was called the Red Sea.

I wake slowly, turn to see if it was all a dream. Her bald head sticks out from under the duvet. Two minutes later, Anna wakes and tries to rub warmth into it. I rub my hot forehead, try to smooth its dull throbbing from last night's whisky. Isla comes in, freezes for just a second, then laughs. Half an hour later Joe does the same, and they both say exactly the same thing.

"Mammy looks funny"

It's what she told them weeks ago. Mammy is going to have medicine that is so strong it will make her hair fall out. And she might look funny for a bit but it will grow back. They giggle further, want to touch her bald head.

"I don't think she looks funny," I say.

But I don't tell them off. Anna told me not to, said it would be their way of dealing with it. It was better than feeling frightened or tearful.

I'm uploading my promotional video and launch recordings to YouTube and Facebook. Anna's outside gardening and the kids are playing out with her. Suddenly the conservatory roof rattles with a door slam. In they come, all three of

201

them, escaping a sudden downpour. Smiles on wet faces. Anna asks them to choose CD's so they can dance and tidy up at the same time. Joe can read. He wants 'rock-star' music, names that sound cool. He gets The Clash, T-Rex, Massive Attack. Isla just picks one within easy reach; Murder Ballads by Nick Cave and the Bad Seeds. They get two songs from each, do far more dancing than tidying. I sit on my computer chair beaming at the three of them, Joe moving like a robot, showing Isla how to break-dance. Anna has her wig on, red headscarf on top, a slim vest top, jeans tucked inside long black leather boots. She looks gorgeous; as good as she's ever looked. Then her and Joe play a game of keep the balloon up and Anna loses the first point because she's too busy trying to tuck her prosthesis back in. I watch them, darting one way then another, under arm and over arm, lunging desperately with feet. All smiles and laughter, even when they're arguing over the score. And it's the most beautiful thing I've seen in my life. And then all goes quiet. Isla goes upstairs and Joe picks up a book. And Anna lies on the floor and does exercises to stop lymphodaema with Joe's plastic lightsaber.

I pick my way over rocks, careful not to step on rubbery strands of seaweed, slicked black around twinkling pools. The others fade further and further behind until I'm way out, calm sea gently swirling and gurgling at my feet. Flat brown seaweed slipping in and out of water like tentacles from a wallowing sea monster. Jimmy said I'd be able to see the caves if I came right out here, if I looked back across at the cliffs. Monks Caves they're called. He used to climb in them as a kid, says he's been inside one further than a mile. They say that one goes all the way to Delaval Hall. Smuggling was a way of life on this North-East coast.

Casks slung beneath the keels of ships. False bottoms in fishing boats. 'Booty' hidden in the holds of ships carrying limestone from Yorkshire to Northumbrian coastal limekilns.

Jimmy comes out. Brings the rest of them. Helen with Arthur and Eleanor, Nic with Owen and Ruby, Anna with Isla and Joe. The rocks are flat and easy this way. The boys jump up and down, pretend they're pirates while adults laugh. But Jimmy's gaze is directed at the cliffs, scanning for that cave of his childhood adventures.

"Loads of us went in there," he says. "You'd come out and there'd be another group just about to go in. It was mint"

Across we go, leaving the rest to return to the beach. We jump from rock to rock, balancing, Jimmy ahead, bristling with anticipation. Twenty years younger. I catch him up just metres from the cliff face, chin in hand.

"It's over on the right, I'm sure it is. That's where we used to climb down, just near the caravan site. We'd come right down the cliff face and make our way across to the cave. There were five or six of us, aged about twelve or thirteen"

He looks across at me, smiles with his whole face.

"We had candles, matches, food. The lot. Two dogs as well. Used to pass them down to each other, then back up again to the cave, half way up the cliff face. A Collie and a Labrador crossed with a Whippet"

And we're picking our way again. Further down where the cliffs turn sharply towards Collywell Bay.

"One time," says Jimmy, "we were inside for hours. And when we came back to the entrance the tide was right in and we had to wait four hours for the sea to move back again. It got dark. And the candles melted ages before we got out. Our hands were covered in wax. This one lad cried

203

for ages, wouldn't stop. We got home about two in the morning. My Mam and Dad were fuming, had called the police and everything. Someone said the council blocked it up not long after that"

We're making our way to two caves and one looks promising. And Jimmy's butterflies are fluttering faster than ever.

"What's that?" I ask, pointing to writing above the first cave.

We jump, balance, occasionally slip our way across. Carved into rock face: W Monk 1904. In we go, a tight diamond shape, sloping downwards.

"This is what it was like," he says. "You'd keep going about eighty feet, then reach a small cave about the size of your bathroom. There was a rope ladder there. You climbed it about twenty feet up and continued. You had to duck most of the way, go in single file, but you'd come to larger caves, different turnings and that"

But this one only goes about thirty feet in. We arrive at the back of it, make our way back out to the sounds of seagulls, the sight of cormorants spreading wings. Then across to a rock fall we go, clamber up giant rocks.

"This is where it is," says Jimmy. "Definitely. The bastards blocked it up"

He looks gutted, talks about getting shovels. How it would only take a few hours. But both of us know we won't. He reckons it's behind all the earth halfway up, behind sprouting grass and delicate purple flowers. We climb further down. Jimmy slumps on a rock, takes tobacco out his back pocket and makes a roll up, all the while looking at this rock fall that's blocking his dreams. That's stopping him from accessing his childhood.

After being away fourteen days I was looking forward to getting back to Ein Yahav. I'd written to my Mam, asked her to send two hundred pounds from my Gran's will to the moshav. It would tide me over a good few weeks in case there wasn't work for a while. But when we got to customs, they refused to let Ray and I enter. We didn't have any money they said. We didn't have flight tickets out. Phone the moshav I said, we have work arranged there. All our belongings are there. I'd been working in Israel five months. We were just having a couple of weeks away in Egypt for a holiday. They weren't interested, remained steadfast, let Claire through though. She felt terrible, hugged us both. Said she'd come back later with the cash my Mam should have sent through. Walked off into Israel. Ray hardly said two words. I argued with Israeli customs for hours. I gave them a phone number for the moshav but they said it didn't work. I was desperate, started to get aggressive. A couple of soldiers were called. They held guns across chests and pushed me backwards. Go back to Egypt they said. Go back to Egypt. We walked back into no man's land. Approached Egyptian customs but they wouldn't have us back either. Back and forth we went, me starting to feel ill and cold, emotional too, like I was about to collapse. Until eventually we were pushed out the Egyptian side and told to go away. We shared a taxi to Taba, the nearest place to the border, a collection of bamboo huts on the beach. And I crashed asleep in the cold with a door that wouldn't close.

Three hours later, I woke up freezing, curled up tight. Then I rushed outside and vomited by the side of the hut. I spent the next hour in the toilets with vomiting and diarrhoea. And when I had nothing left to throw up I spat stomach lining and blood. Then I staggered back to the hut, all aches and pains, to tell a sleepy Ray there was something wrong with me. When I collected the energy we got the bus to Sharm el-Sheikh. And then we waited four a half hours for the bus to Cairo. I climbed into my sleeping bag, my head pounding. Looked out the window as we drove through the night. My body shook as I remembered my first three and a half months in Israel. As valleys and mountains floated through my mind, suffused with the aroma of falling in love.

PART VII

I leave Isla in bed with her Mammy, head under duvet talking to her knees, drive through mists to work. Radio 4 tells of expense claims by MP's, stacks them up, explains there's more to come. Holiday cottage renovations, wreaths, light bulb fitting, ornamental duck ponds, dog food, moats and helipads. Second homes in South London when they have a first in North. I park up, walk past dozens of prison officers and talk of strike.

In the classroom I'm taking prisoners through Games People Play, relating it to characters and writing in general. I'm explaining how people's interactions are often "a patterned and predictable series of transactions which are superficially plausible but actually conceal motivations and lead to a well-defined predictable outcome." And I'm trying to explain how this could be useful in both understanding people and creating characters with depth. But then a student interrupts.

"Look," he says. "I'm not being funny. I understand what you're doing here and why you're doing it. But this isn't what I'm here for. If I wanted psychology I'd go on a fucking psychology course"

I'm stumped. Don't know what to say. I've been told by a number of prisoners what they think of psychologists. They begrudge the impact they have upon their lives and sentences. Say they're so young they don't have enough experience of life. State they're always looking for signs of further offending or denial. Twist words to suit aims.

He looks at me a few seconds, then carries on, embarrassed by my silence.

"It's not that it can't help, this kind of stuff. But listen to what this man said"

Jabs his thumb towards the man on his left.

"He's trying to block some things out. He told you that ten minutes ago. I think this is a bit too deep for some people in here, not the right time for them. You can open doors for them and then, you know, things could happen later on"

I stutter for a couple of seconds. Then talk about the difficulty of finding the balance, that worrying too much about opening doors could mean diluting everything. That opening doors can release the best kind of writing. That I hadn't asked anyone to contribute anything personal and had simply talked generally about particular games. But yes, perhaps I should be more aware of where I am, though it was always my intention to treat students as normal people within the classroom.

We have a class discussion about it and there's a split. Four think the material is too deep, three think it's useful and one hasn't been paying any attention.

A big clump of Anna's hair has appeared in the middle of the back garden. Its dark form stands out against sunlit grass, curled together like a Marx brother's wig. Like a hedgehog with a perm. I ask Anna what it's doing there. She says she found it down the side of the bench. Put it out this morning in case the birds wanted to make a nest of it. Then she talks about the future, for her and her breasts. Or lack of them. Ever since she felt that lump that turned out to be a cyst, she's decided she doesn't want to live a life paranoid of returning cancer. Before the mastectomy she said she'd have a reconstruction. Joked if she got both off together she'd get a bigger pair, then decided she'd be happy with just being perked up a bit. Recently though, she's been doubtful.

"They're ten hour operations," she says. "And I won't be able to get both of them done together"

I smile.

"I'll support you either way. You know that, don't you?"

She does. And perhaps that, added to the fact she's emotionally stable, means she doesn't feel pressured to have breasts return to her body. I'm proud of her. I really am; how she can take decisions based on individual circumstance rather than societal pressure. And I will support her either way. I'll love her and find her attractive whatever she chooses. But I'm only human. And I'm prone to shallowness at times. I'd prefer her to have breasts rather than not.

Anna's quieter than usual this morning. I finish my coffee, read Isla a book. Anna's just started to sit up for her cup of tea, has hardly said a word. Today is chemo day, the second of six, and she's going by herself, insists upon it. I leave her lying there, go down the harbour with Caffrey. The swans have returned. They sit silently, heads arced towards water. Scanning for fishes pushed along by the smooth tide. Across the water a young man sits on a bench. Legs clamped together, arms tight around waist. Collar up and head down, hat pulled tight all the way over. He doesn't move, looks like he's been there all night, like he's trying to blot out the new day and all it brings. We walk right past him, sitting there as if paralysed, oblivious to cars that roar like waves on the bridge above him. And then we leave him behind and go down the dene where we're welcomed by blackbird song, the coo of rock pigeons and crowing of cockerels, where leaves wave in the breeze, creating their own light show on pink campion, stitchwort and cow parsley.

"Sticky kiss test," says Isla, climbing on my knee. She puts a hand on my shoulder, purses her lips. I kiss her marmite and marmalade moustache. Pull a face and pretend it was horrible. She throws her head back, bursts out laughing. I cuddle her, look out the window, notice the hedgehog with a perm is still there. Then I make my breakfast and listen to MP's saying their expenses were "within the rules." The next story tells me unemployment has risen to 2.2 million. Two hundred and eighty thousand people have lost their jobs in the first three months of the year. Things are going to get worse.

This week's donation tally stands at one rhubarb crumble, one bottle of elderberry wine, homemade soup, lettuce, spinach and plants for the garden, all from Lin. A bottle of fortified wine from Les, a Thornton's chocolate cake, a packet of giant chocolate buttons and a packet of raspberry ruffles from Noelene. Then there's homemade quiche, scones and cakes from Ellen. I look down at my belly that I never had to worry about until the last few years. I make the pledge to do more exercise yet again, wonder if I should take the donations into work. Then I eat a cake and have some chocolate buttons to get a bit more energy for writing.

We got into Cairo at five in the morning. Took a taxi to the Oxford Hotel. Crashed in reception until nine, then went to Thomas Cook who told me their flights back to England were £200 and it wasn't possible to reverse charges from Egypt. I needed to get home to my Mam in Hartlepool, to see my girl in Newcastle if she still was my girl. And so I walked to the British Embassy but it was closed for two days. Then, when the hotel owner found Ray and myself had only ten pounds between us, he took our passports so we couldn't leave without paying. As for my illness; diarrhoea came in muddy waves. Sickness in erratic explosions. But there were increasing moments in between when I just felt weak. I stayed in the hotel as much as I could, did nothing. Noise outside pounded my head. The usual city chaos turned my guts. Someone let me share a few joints and I had this waking nightmare that my immune system had closed down after being attacked by HIV. I listened to talk about adventure, was desperate to get home. Then back to my room where Ray said nothing.

And I wanted to say to him, "Just for once Ray, please laugh. Please say something funny. I'm stoned and I feel really bad and I need to laugh but I can't do it by myself." After another day of doing nothing and eating nothing I tried the Embassy again. They wouldn't let me use their phone but said I could reverse charges in Egypt, would have to find the Communications Centre to set it up. When I found the Communications Centre they told me it was impossible to make reverse charge calls. After insisting and being bundled between desks and arguing with two people they said okay, but not from there. By this time I was so upset at constantly banging my head against a wall for something that should have been so easy I burst into tears and made my way back to the Oxford. Someone suggested the Hilton. And so I went there, conspicuous in filthy clothes, scruffy beard and ill pallor - but way past caring. Half an hour of frustration followed but then, when I heard a ring tone and my Mam answered, I couldn't speak for crying.

I'm on my way to be interviewed by Laura, who works for Isolationist and New Writing North. I'm trying to work out how many copies I need to sell just to break even. £3.80 for the metro. A couple of quid for the petrol to the metro station. £4.00 for a cup of coffee to wake me up and a bottle of sparkling water so my mouth doesn't dry up. Fifteen per cent per copy is about £1.20 each, presuming they buy it full price even though there are plenty already at less than half. That means I need to sell eight copies from this interview just to break even. But then Laura arrives, and she's lovely and interested. And she's read half the book and is enjoying it. And I'm sat here, while Anna is in hospital having chemotherapy pumped into her bloodstream. And someone's talking to me like I really am a writer, and I'm loving it. I tell her I want to make a living out of writing, not just my own but others too. Like any new writer I dream about bestsellers, being flown abroad, put up in swish hotels. But it's not just my stories I want to tell. I want to help others write their stories, get them published too. That's why I'm in prison teaching creative writing. I want to work with Victim Support too, in mental health settings, palliative care. With estranged fathers and the elderly. I want to capture stories before their owners leave this world. I tell Laura about this old man I worked with last year, in a hostel for homeless men with mental health problems. They said he wouldn't speak to me. His best friend died two weeks earlier. He'd watched it happen, was still traumatised by it. He wouldn't move out the kitchen where the death happened unless he had to. I sat with him half an hour before either of us spoke. I watched him roll and smoke one cigarette after the other. Crack open a can of cheap lager. Dribble it down his grey stubble chin. Then, after all that silence, he pointed towards the kitchen sink.

"It was over there. That's where it happened"

I nodded.

"Blood started coming out his nose. Pouring on the floor. We were just sat here having a drink that's all. Then all of a sudden he stood up and out it came, pouring all over the floor"

I kept quiet and so he continued.

"I shouted at him. We were both hammered, had been drinking all day. I shouted, 'get yourself over to the sink man. You're making a mess all over the floor. Get over to the sink.' He grabbed a mop that was leaning against that cupboard, started trying to mop all the blood up. Then he just collapsed on the floor and died right in front of us, the blood pouring out of him like a tap"

He talked the next four hours non-stop, told me about his life in the merchant navy. What the ships were like, the people he worked with. How he'd visited America and Japan, been all over the Far East. His stories were fascinating, full of characters and adventure. I'd be surprised if he were alive now. But I was delighted to have heard part of his story. And I think it may have helped him, if only for that day, that he had someone to listen to it.

Anna's immunity is low. Much lower than it should be. They weren't going to give her the chemo, had to check it out with the doctor. Just this once he said. Never again. I turn the radio off, don't want Anna to hear it; a programme on breast cancer and screening. It's followed a woman through the process, is at the results stage. I get a lump myself, except this one's in my stomach. Her results are negative. I picture her smile, hear that great big sigh of relief. Then Anna walks in and tells me about her immunity so I turn it off and my lump disappears. I want to tell her I have a half hour radio slot coming up on Resonance FM, a respected arts and culture radio station with forty thousand listeners. It could make a difference, send my book to the next level. But Anna tells me her neutrophils, the immune system's white blood cells, are down to 1.2. The cut off is 1.5. It will be the only time the doctor gives the go-ahead if her immunity remains that low. I don't really understand what she's talking about. But I do know she has to be extremely careful not to catch any infection or germ. She says anything, even a rise in temperature, means having to be rushed into hospital immediately. I nod my head, look out into the back garden. The permed hedgehog has gone, probably blown into someone else's garden. But who knows, maybe there's a proud bird out there, showing off his new nest to his neighbours. Anna says the chemo is kicking in already. We sit down for tea and she can feel her taste buds going as she eats each mouthful. The sickness is coming on too. Then we're finished and there's a moment. So I tell her about Resonance. She goes up to the calendar, shouts from the kitchen.

"Its two days after my fifth chemotherapy. There couldn't be a worse time"

"Well you haven't written it down," I snap.

She walks back in with the calendar, shows me a little red c.

"I wrote it small because there's a chance it could be changed or put back"

"Aaahh..."

Then silence for a moment until Anna adds someone else to the mixer.

"And it's right by Louise's due date too, so if I'm not able to look after the kids I can't ask her or my brother either"

I sigh like a petulant child.

"I won't go then"

"Don't worry," she says. "I'll get someone to come and help me"

"I'll change the date. It's not confirmed yet"

"No really, it doesn't matter"

"Of course it matters"

She won't budge. Says I could change the date and then her chemo might be put back anyway. It's important. I should just do it. We put the kids to bed after telly. She sits on the couch and reads a magazine. I do some research on the internet for my students. They had a debate over when and why trousers were invented, came up with all sorts of suggestions. I find they were invented by nomads of Central Asia to stop chafing, around three thousand years ago. Consequently the Romans saw them as barbaric and banned them for hundreds of years.

I call my Mam. She's trying to move to a healthier environment but has had no interest in her house. And they've had to rule out the whole of Lanchester because it's dangerous to live within three miles of a radio or TV mast. She tells me of the danger of cordless phones, mobile phones too, anything that's electrical but doesn't involve cables. How the electrical pulses damage the energy in your body. She has a mobile phone but its turned off, used only for emergencies, occasional texting. I nod my head. Continue speaking on our cordless phone, sat at my wireless laptop with my mobile phone in my trouser pocket.

After one more day hanging about the Oxford Hotel, of meals of dry bread and water, I went to Barclays and was given money sent by my Mam. I went back to the hotel

216

relieved to find Ray, who was going every day to the Irish Embassy as they'd told him they would get in touch with his Mam and would receive money there if she was able to send any. I'd decided to go to the airport and try to get a standby flight. Ray wanted me to stay another four or five days but I was desperate to get out. I booked a plane for that night, though it wasn't direct. It was with Romanian Airways and included a six hour wait in Bucharest. I didn't care, just needed to get moving again. I felt guilty telling Ray then avoided all offered joints. My last hour at the Oxford Hotel was spent listening to Emo tell how he'd walked on all the planets and Pluto was the best. I left at ten p.m., gave Ray a hug, told him to keep in touch but somehow knew that neither of us would. The last argument with a taxi driver was almost enjoyable. And then there was one last stumbling block. The guard at the airport wouldn't believe the picture on my passport was me. I explained I was fifteen years old on the picture but was now twenty-two. Had dreadlocks and a beard instead of bum fluff. Eventually a manager let me board the plane and, after a weak cup of tea, a rubbery cheese sandwich and a six hour wait in cold Bucharest, I touched down in London and had my rucksack turned over. The next day I got the bus up to Hartlepool and my loving mother was waiting at the station for me.

I kiss her face as soon as my eyes open, although I get the impression she's been awake for some time. She looks serene. Taking away hair hasn't made her look masculine.

It's emphasised her feminine features instead. But she's been wearing her headscarf at night to stop her head getting too cold.

I pull back, get some distance.

"You looks classy," I tell her.

She gives me a funny look.

"You do," I insist. "You look like that film with your headscarf on, that painting. The girl with the pearl earring"

She smiles.

"I feel like a girl from another planet"

Then it's downstairs for breakfast because the kids can't wait another second. Though Isla finds little time to eat, she's talking so much. Conversations include cardigans and whether she's got one or two, her best friends Sarah, Eden and Ester, the colour of Mrs Dale's jumper, whether Mrs Lawless has been off school because she's poorly or just because she's sitting at home watching telly, tights, swimming lessons, the pouring rain outside and the fact that Heather, two years older and who gave Isla her school cardigan, won't let her be her best friend unless she lies on her side with her head on the grass.

Creeping mists suffocate the drone of fog-horn, over hard pale sands pushed tight by waves. Tangled in fishing line, slapped down by seaweed, old buoys and beer cans, a little pink teddy lies face down in sand. I stoop and feel its salt soaked fur while its one eye looks back at me from a battered face. Picking it up, I wonder how it arrived here, if it came from over the North Sea. A visitor from Scandinavia? Or hurled from the pier by a lover deceived? Maybe it came from the railings half a mile up the coast. A little girl murdered by waves and rocks. I sit it down gently, looking half out to sea, imagine a dog cocking its leg. Toss it back in again. Let fate determine where it will travel, who may find it next.

Isla climbs over, sticks her knee in my face, gets under the duvet and grins. Her Mammy doesn't move, has her back turned to us. Isla says "tickle tickle" and stretches out fingers to the bald head sticking out. Still no movement. So Isla climbs over the top of her Mammy's pillow, curls her body around the top of her head like a cat. Peers at her closed eyes. She wants attention, hasn't seen her Mammy since yesterday morning. Eventually Anna turns round and smiles. Isla kisses her on the mouth and laughs. Can't stop still for more than two seconds. Anna turns away again, reaches for the anti-nausea tablets. Says having Isla in the bed is like being at sea.

I take Caffrey out, meet Wilf in the shop, walk back with him, papers in hand. He asks how Anna is so I tell him about cancer, about chemotherapy. He must have been the only person in the street not to know. He tells me about his wife having breast cancer. She got over it, two years later went to the dentist because her gums were hurting. Had cancer there too. They took a rib out of her, used it to construct a new jawbone. She was only out the weekend, had to go straight back in again. Spent six weeks in intensive care. That's as far as his story goes. We've reached our house. He sends his love to Anna, goes on his way. I wonder how much longer his wife lived, whether it was days or years. There's just him and his son these days, has been for the six years we've lived in the street.

Anna didn't get any sleep at all last night. She laid as still as a corpse, heard the sounds of piano being played. Chemotherapy can exaggerate schizophrenic tendencies, she says. Then she started thinking about crackers and cheese, how beautiful they would taste. Couldn't get the image out of her mind. Eventually she got up, made some but they tasted terrible. So she took a hot chocolate out into the garden. Sat in starlight serenity with the plants and flowers stretching up to the moon.

I sit at the table, separate sections of newspaper. Turn instantly to football. Read about Manchester United's eighteenth league title. Smile at how I didn't even think about the review section, realise I might as well get it over with. So I flick through the pages; three paperbacks reviewed and I'm not one of them. Then Anna comes in from the back garden, is worried about an injured bird outside. Has taken it some crumbs. I'm more interested in the football but she keeps talking about it. I turn my head, see it slumped on the step. It struggles about ten inches, puts its head on a piece of wood. Stays there. Breathes slowly but doesn't move otherwise. Anna tells Joe. I return to the football.

"What kind of bird is it?" asks Joe.

"A blackbird," says Anna. "A *Mammy* blackbird"

The word pricks my head up. I look at Anna and Joe. Her putting make up on, spreading it higher than ever, up over her forehead where hair once was. Him peering out the window.

"Are we going to bury it?" he asks.

I decide to check for cats.

"Yes," says Anna, then smiles a second. "But we'll wait for it to die first"

The receptionist looked concerned when I asked how I could get in touch with one of the student nurses. She wouldn't tell me where their accommodation was, then eventually said if I hung around I might see some of them coming back. I walked back out the grand entrance of the Royal Victoria Infirmary, sat down on the statue of Queen Victoria. Gazed at the bright yellow flowerbed directly in front. Then, after a quick check, I went and helped myself to a bouquet. Twenty minutes later she came walking down the path, back from the supermarket with five bags of shopping. All by herself. Browner than she was in Israel. I jumped off Queen Victoria and walked across, bouquet behind back. She gave a quick glance, then looked away again, more concerned with the heaviness of her bags. Half a second later her head twisted my way once more. Her look wasn't one of delight, the flooding relief of a wife whose husband has returned from the war. It was one of incomprehension. Of sheer bewilderment.

"I...I thought you were in Egypt?"

I beamed as wide as my mouth would allow.

"I was"

Then my arm came from behind and produced the bunch of stolen daffodils.

She smiled for the first time, but still with a look of disbelief. Half shrugged. We didn't embrace; she had too many bags and was too shocked. Had spent months getting used to the fact I wasn't with her, may never be with her. I swapped the flowers for a few bags.

"Come on then. Let's put the shopping away"

Through the corridors of the RVI we went, hardly talking, until we came to the nurses' accommodation at the far end. She took me to her small room, a double bed taking up half the available space, posters all over walls. One small window that looked out to the front of the hospital. Put her flowers in a tiny sink. Took the bags from me.

"I'll put the shopping away. You better stay here. We're not allowed visitors"

And then she left. I looked around, found the shalom poster from Jerusalem. Spiralled shells in a bowl. Other mementoes trapped in a tiny space. She came back with someone else, introduced her new best friend Jane. Said later she was in such shock she didn't know what to say, needed someone with her. Half an hour later Jane disappeared and Anna and I had our first cuddle for months. We chatted and rolled our first ever joint together. Smoked it out the window. Looked down at the statue of Queen Victoria, the daffodil flower bed. I breathed cannabis into my lungs and my head started to fill up, my brain spin. It permeated throughout me, turned my thoughts internal, made me feel claustrophobic. Anna turned and did something inside. I stayed rooted to the spot. This wasn't how I'd dreamt it would be. I glanced back but returned my gaze through the window, felt compelled to look out into open space. When Rob left Afiq we had a house to ourselves, albeit a small one. We had valleys and seas, beaches and ancient cities. Adventure and exploration. And now we had a room ten feet square that looked out onto a statue, a small garden. Then a wall. Reality sank into my bones. And for the first time since before that night I crashed my bike into the hedge and we kissed on the grass, I wondered if she was the right girl for me. I stared out the window, heard her rustling behind. Thought maybe it really was just an extended holiday romance brought about by excitement, by travel and sunshine.

I finish reading Ben 10, help Joe choose three books for himself in bed, hear David's deep voice as I'm coming downstairs. But I see the back of Anna's bald head before I see him or his fiancée Christine. It's not working out how I thought it would, this baldness. It's like she's determined to show off her new enforced style. This is me. Get used to it. I'm okay with it and I want you to be too. I never expected her to be like this, however many times she said she wasn't bothered about losing her hair, that it was about living - and if baldness was a stage towards life then so be it. She plays it safe in one way though, only revealing herself to close friends. And she hasn't gone alfresco at school yet. Says she's too concerned that others will feel awkward, won't know what to say. Doesn't want to freak the kids out.

She's still trying to get children to decide what they want for breakfast. Joe settles for toast with four different spreads. I walk into the kitchen, look at Anna.

"Do you want me to do it?"

"Yes I do"

She cuts two slices of bread like she's trying to cut her fingers off.

"It's quarter past eight. They need to get sorted, have their breakfast"

"I know. That's what I'm going to do"

She reaches down into the bottom cupboard. Takes out her makeup bag. Doesn't look at me. I take honey and marmite out the cupboard, stare at her while she pours herself a cup of tea. And then she glares back. "Am I not allowed to be angry?" She doesn't actually say it out loud but that's what her look says. I realise I do that so much of the time. Justify my own moods when I'm in them. Think they should be respected and accepted as part of me. But when Anna's in a mood, which happens far less often, then I find it a challenge, a threat. And I'm up for an argument. I'm out to justify my own position instead of respecting someone else's.

Anna's outside, taking seedlings to the greenhouse, making use of the last hour of sunlight. She tells me she hasn't slept for five nights now. Not a wink. Feels like she's on amphetamines. She knows her body's shattered but her mind is wired and won't stop working, won't let her relax. It's the steroids, the tablets she takes to stop the nausea. The alternative is to not take the steroids and bring the sickness back. Sickness or sleep? They're the choices. She decides she'll try and find a balance. Take half the steroids only. Have a little bit of both.

The boiler man spends far more time talking to me than he does checking and fixing our boiler. He's not able to stop once he's started, swinging from topic to topic. From youths these days to caravans and his son being a Butlins redcoat. From how men shouldn't wear earrings to having three other customers who are writers. I stand there, nod my head, feign interest when I desperately want to get on the computer and get writing. Anna comes back from taking the kids to school and I tell her that's the last time she arranges for him to come round while I'm home alone. It happened last time too. I don't mind if others are at home but Wednesdays and Friday mornings are my only free times to write.

Anna looks indignant.

"I booked him for now because I didn't know how I'd be feeling, if I'd be well enough"

She makes some breakfast, calls the hospital. Has developed a rash over much of her upper torso, probably provoked by steroids.

"I'm taking antihistamines to stop the side effects of the steroids which I'm taking to stop the side effects of the chemo," she says.

Then she shows me her hands. They've gone a dark brown colour. The chemo makes her much more sensitive to the sun. The hospital wanted her to pop in but she says she feels okay, is sure it's the steroids. Is sick of appointments all the time. Agrees to go straight to Accident and Emergency if she gets a temperature. The rest of her hair is coming out too, though her eyelashes and eyebrows are proving stubborn, much to her approval. She's hardly any hair on her arms now, very little pubic hair left either. In fact the only hair that may not fall out is on her legs, the only hair she'd like to lose.

That week was among the greatest of my life. I turned round from the window and took hold of her. We stayed in bed for much of the next four or five days, smoked lots of joints, had lots of sex. Occasionally Anna lifted herself to go to college. Once we even went as far as getting the metro to Tynemouth with Jane and her boyfriend, drank champagne and had piggy back fights. And then we got the train to Hartlepool and my parents fell in love with Anna too, as I knew they would. But apart from that, the only other time we left the bed was to tiptoe around the hospital corridors at night. Trying to find the vending machine and cure our munchies, but not wake anyone official who would realise I was an intruder.

After a few weeks though, it was time to be travelling again. I had belongings, money, clothes, a tent I'd never unrolled in the Negev Desert. So I decided to use my last will money to fly to Israel, collect my belongings, get the ferry to a Greek Island to find work. After all, that was the plan before Israeli customs and amoebic dysentery got in the way. And I couldn't stay in the RVI as I wasn't allowed to be there in the first place. I hugged Anna goodbye and we cried once more. She promised to come and see me in Greece. I hugged my parents, went down to London, stayed a few nights then hugged my friends. Boarded a flight to Tel Aviv, stayed the night there. Met an English man who could juggle and play Captain Pugwash on the harmonica at the same time. A Chilean man who walked on his hands to add to the entertainment. I worked as an extra in a television advert for the Likud's general election campaign, put on blue clothes with two hundred other travellers and soldiers. Formed the Star of David and waved whilst being videoed from the air. Whilst there I met two girls called Sam and Lorraine who were also going to Greece. We arranged to meet at Haifa after I picked my money and belongings up from the moshav.

When I got to Ein Yahav Gary seemed surprised to see me. And when I mentioned Claire his mood changed for the worst. Two hours later a furious Claire walked in with friends, accused Gary of throwing away her belongings. An argument ensued and although Gary denied everything vehemently it became rather obvious he'd dumped her belongings when she went off to Egypt without him. Then, when I walked into my old room and began to ask questions and root around, I realised things of mine were missing too. No shells I'd collected with Anna. Clothes missing. No tape from Anna. No chocolates from Hester and no money from my Mam though she told me she'd sent it for my return from Egypt. I had sixty pounds to my name. Wasn't able to get anymore. Again, Gary denied everything. Someone else had stayed for a few days he said. Claire searched his room with me present but nothing turned up. And so I collected what I did have and took it all to Claire's house instead.

What is it about the sight and sound of water? The feel too? It draws me, especially now, hung over from last night's warming performances from Baloa and The Week That Was. I cross rippled contours, walk to where waves come slowly gliding in, marble reflecting the new day's sunshine. Caffrey scares a group of gulls into taking off. They skim the sea before landing on rocks further out. Mine are the only human footprints out here, next to Caffrey's paw prints and the pointed arrows of bird feet. I lift my feet away, watch water rising up from under the surface. To my left, channels run back to their mother, past sand that blows tiny baby bubbles. Broken shells that glisten like trickery. An hour later and I'm back on the beach with the rest of the family. Anna hovers by the soft dry sand. I take Isla and Joe's hands and we charge into the sea, shoes and socks off, trousers rolled up. We splash around, look at each other with open mouths. It cools the head as well as the heels; natures reflexology. Jumping waves and kicking up splashes we're soon a hundred metres away, Anna a tiny figure sat down by the harbour entrance. And then I realise my trainers were left by the water.

"Come on," I shout. "The tide's coming in"

Off we run, the three of us. Sending up spray, checking ahead. Hands flat like peaked caps to block the sun.

"They're out at sea," points Joe. "They're floating away"

He runs on laughing, then realises it's only seaweed. And then he sees something moving in the water around his ankles and screams. A couple of crabs legs tumble over and over, claw over claw. I pick up the line that's attached to them, that's wound them, bound them together. Explain it's not a mutant crab, just legs entangled. I swing them round in circles but that causes more screams so I hold them still and pull the line. The other end is stuck in sand. The children gather round, fascinated at where it's gone. I pull harder and harder and eventually it slides out. A beautiful weight shaped like a fish. Green and yellow glittering scales and a staring eyeball. Deadly three pronged hook with barbs attached.

We left bars and restaurants, walked up through the old town. Past stone buildings that clutched pink flowers to crumbling walls. Old women with beady eyes in front of whitewashed apartments. Buildings gave way to fields, small street to uneven track. We looked up at the mountain, glanced behind to check we weren't being watched. Stepped behind trees into an onion field. I threw my rucksack and tent onto the ground, stretched my back.

An hour later, I spread my thin foam mat down, laid on top of it. Shuffled about and groaned while Sam and Lorraine giggled.

"I don't know what you two are laughing about. At least I've got something to sleep on"

We'd had fun on the ferry, got drunk and slept outside. Spent a night in Rhodes then carried on to Crete. Malia was where the work was because that's where the English tourists went. Sam and Lorraine got jobs within three days. Bar and restaurant owners were male, liked pretty girls working for them. I trawled everywhere with no success. Eventually, Sam sorted a job for me, meeting tourists in Iraklion for an airline company. But when I went to see the boss he wouldn't employ me. I was too scruffy, had dreadlocks. And so I queued up with Albanians early the next morning for work picking potatoes. You had to fill seven sacks to make a pound. But they didn't pick me when the truck came along and I was left standing while most climbed in and drove off. And then, that same night, a DJ from a new nightclub due to open said I could be his light and sound man, but when I went along the next day his manager wouldn't give me a job either. Sam and Lorraine started to get annoyed at staying in the tent. I figured they wanted to move out into an apartment but felt guilty leaving me. I had to meet them both after work, walk them home in the dark. Out the village and up the lane. Through trees and into a bumpy onion field to our tent with no light and no water. Where we slept with the ants, with mosquitoes and lizards.

And then English lads and lasses started to arrive by the plane load. Football tops and heaving bosoms. Sloshing down pints and suggestive dancing. And my hopes at finding work increased as the bars and nightclubs started to fill. I wrote to Anna each night, sent a letter every week, not knowing if she was getting my letters, desperate for her to come and see me as promised but knowing money would be difficult to find. Someone called Steve turned up and squeezed into the tent. The girls knew him from Dahab in Egypt. But Lorraine found out her Grandfather died so her and Sam flew back to England just four weeks after we'd arrived. I couldn't afford the bus fare to see them off as I'd spent most my money on cheap retsina wine. Either that or waiting round bars for a boss to turn up. Steve paid me on. In the end the four of us spent three nights sleeping outside Iraklion airport until the girls could get a charter flight home. And then back to the tent I went, sharing with just Steve, my clothes filthy as I couldn't afford laundry. Salvation almost came in the form of Marco, a 54 year old white haired Irish guy who'd slept on the beach for the past twelve years after splitting up with his wife. Some said he was a member of the IRA and on the run but I wasn't so sure. Anyway, he'd found someone who wanted to buy an English passport for three hundred pounds. But the buyer, who looked Chinese, decided to plump for someone else's instead. I cursed my bad luck, not even able to make money illegally. Left Marco with his new best friend Victor, a Yugoslavian who'd slept on the beach with him the last three months. Victor had run away from the war, was easily spotted because of a green baseball cap he never took off, even when he went to sleep. One morning he showed me why. Removed it slowly. Three bullet holes had been put in his head. A plastic sheet was attached with bolts on either side where his skull had been blown away. And then Steve left too, back to England as both his sisters were due to give birth. I hugged him goodbye and returned to my tent in the onion field, alone.

I come back from work to find Garrard, a friend since school days, with Heather and their two children Jacob and Holly. Joe and Jacob are running wild in the garden, refusing to listen, wired to their own beat. They come in for tea but can't stop still, can't keep quiet. Can't even eat they're so excited. Two hours later the adults sit round the same table, dulled by lack of sleep and an overabundance of cajoling and repetition. Two years ago we'd have been half cut by now. The language would have been flowing with wit and laughter, sarcastic put downs and the latest music. We'd have been in the living room on the couch or rug but that seems too comfy tonight. Better the hard wooden chairs and a table to keep yourself propped up on. We sit and chat, smile and yawn. The bottle of whisky stays in the kitchen, untouched. Joe and Jacob are wide awake upstairs, studying a pile of books to keep them quiet, acres of free disc space in their minds. Holly is wandering around, unable to settle. We won't manage three bottles of wine between the four of us but at least we're still together. And how lucky we are too; both with beautiful children, one of each. An older brother to look after a younger sister or get annoyed at her hanging around with him and his mates. As time passes, life seems to open out into a series of stages. Of challenges. Here we are, Anna and I, our friends kept alongside as we've all grown up, mid-thirties to forty. The stage of striving to keep relationships together with young children running and screaming. Shouting and sighing. Struggling and juggling with something we never thought would be so all encompassing, so joyful but also so tiring and repetitive at times. And we're the lucky ones. For there are those that haven't managed to keep that spark, have grown weary and separated. Suspicion and anger muscling in to deal with divorce and houses. Access to children. And those that haven't had children, who are striving to fulfil dreams and expectations before it's too late. Fearful that nature has played a cruel trick on them but kept silent all along. It's the stage of parents becoming elderly too. Their hands curling as lines grow deeper and tighten. Heading towards heaven or soil. To be scattered on waves or mountains. It's the stage to speak about those issues that have lain dormant. That have moved further below the surface as the winds of time have covered them with more earth. Heather rises to blow her double lilo up with a hairdryer. I show Caffrey the back door and look away when his pleading eyes ask for more.

My sister calls to say the five of them have a cold. They'll not be able to come over because of the risk to Anna. Joe's hugely disappointed at not seeing Jasmine and her younger sisters. He adores his time with them. But Anna's immunity has fallen to 0.4. She can't risk getting a virus or it's straight to hospital for an intravenous drip. Her immunity needs to be up to 1.5 in three days' time or they won't give her the chemo. It would be her third out of six as well; halfway there. And her right breast has become infected where the central line tunnels into flesh.

It seems there's a pattern emerging. Anna has her headscarf on when in the back garden, her wig and headscarf on when going out the front door and any combination of those two and bald head when inside. Sometimes I have a conversation with her and she's got hair. Then I pick something up or put something away. And when I turn round again she's bald.

He can't stop reading, Joe. He has at least one hour with his books every night. And that's just official time. We tread carefully up stairs, careful not to creak, catch him at it every night. Sneaky reading with the bedside light on. You could probably storm up the stairs shouting and he wouldn't scramble for the light though, he gets so absorbed. You have to walk right up to him, say his name five times, lean over and switch the light off, remind him its bedtime. And it's not just night time either. He doesn't stop wherever he goes. Street signs. Shop names. Peering over my shoulder at the computer when he says goodnight, mouth moving to the rhythm. What was once a source of frustration has turned into something far more compelling. He's been on year two books now for months, though he's still in year one. He flies through them with ease, hardly stopping to take a breath. In many other situations he finds it hard to concentrate. He's a dreamer like his Daddy, is floating somewhere else. But when it comes to books he can sit there for hours oblivious to all else. Focus and escape into a different world.

I don't know what compelled me to check the post as I walked down to my new job that morning. Some serious looking woman handed over a letter with Anna's handwriting on and I read it walking to work. She was flying to Iraklion, had nowhere to stay. Nothing but a return flight and very little money. From there, she planned to get a bus to Malia and walk around the bars showing a photo of me. She didn't know if I'd got a job or had moved from Malia searching for work elsewhere, but she desperately hoped I would get this letter. Her flight was due in that very afternoon. I spent the day as assistant chef at Malia Beach Bar, slightly amusing considering I couldn't cook, left early and got the bus to Iraklion. Her flight was ten hours late, would arrive in the middle of the night. I bought a bottle of retsina, set the alarm on my watch and crashed out on the grass. When the alarm went off I washed my face in the toilets, put the wildflowers I'd picked into the empty retsina bottle and waited at arrivals.

Anna stayed for two weeks. The first thing she did was buy two lilos for the tent. Then she met my new friends but on the second night a Northern Irish lad called Jammo was arrested and jailed for eight months for punching a bar owner who'd groped his girlfriend. So Anna spent the next few nights walking around with a bucket as we had to raise two thousand pounds to buy him out. We managed to raise four hundred and his friend came out with the rest. Anna lounged about in the day time while I worked. I put sun beds out at nine a.m., swam a hundred metres out to sea and back again to wake up. Had freshly squeezed orange and strong black coffee. Worked in the kitchens cooking burgers and washing up. Stalios the chef gave Anna free alcohol and food. Scouser Rich and I stood inside the kitchen, drank a few pints, smoked cigarettes. Listened to Stalios tell about his six girlfriends in six different places whilst waiting for the lunchtime rush. And every so often when it wasn't too busy I went outside and sat with Anna in the sun. On the night we went out and got drunk, accepted free drinks from friends who worked in bars. Then we staggered back to my tent in the onion field. But after two weeks Anna flew back to Newcastle. I watched her walk away from me at the airport. She didn't look back, just carried straight on. I turned away, drank a bottle of retsina and slept on the grass until morning.

Jammo came out of prison a few days after Anna left. We held a party for him. He couldn't stop smiling. Drank himself drunk and then sober again. Said jail was full of Albanians but they didn't cause him any bother. The next week I got my first letter from Anna since she'd been over on holiday. She'd thought it over, wasn't happy studying to be a nurse anymore. She'd started working in a pub in the Bigg Market. Would do as many shifts as possible to save whatever money she could. Then, after three months, she was coming out to join me. I folded the letter in my hands, closed my eyes, leant back, breathed in air that suddenly seemed much sweeter. All I had to do she said was keep my job. Keep my job, save as much money as possible and let her know where I'd be in November.

It's June already. The weeks are sliding by. It's nearly five months since Anna discovered that first lump in the shower. It's halfway through the year, nearly halfway through chemotherapy. Nobody could ever have imagined this would happen as they woke up on New Year's Day and wondered about the year ahead. Our dreams and New Year resolutions didn't involve fighting cancer, the possibility of death. I drive to work in glorious sunshine, listen to Michael Howard and Alistair Darling being put under pressure for expense claims, Susan Boyle being escorted to The Priory by police officers after a mental health assessment. My teaching is leaden. I didn't prepare properly and the class are bored.

The afternoon class is quite the opposite though. My most prolific writer's in this class. But he's having one of those doubtful moments most writers surely have. He's used to sniggering from other prisoners, to those who think he's a crackpot with just another conspiracy theory. That doesn't bother him. And he's as convinced as ever that his theories are true. He's just wondering if all the work will be worth it, if the book will be successful, get people talking. He doesn't care about money he says. He cares about turning the world round, about helping people see how secret powers are driving us forwards into a one world state. This book has been his crutch for six years, though he's been investigating its issues for thirty. Others in prison turn to religion, to drugs. Sink into depression. But writing's his daily fix and he can't get it out his system. Then there's talk of Trinidad, Antigua. Beach life. Noise and vitality. Passion and beautiful women. A student asks if I ever get to the beach. I let slip a little something of my life. It's frowned upon in such an establishment. I say I've got a dog, walk him every morning, every night, often in the middle of the day too. I have beach, cliffs and dene within a few minutes' walk. It gets my creative juices going, de-stresses me. I turn back to the man who asked me, ten years my junior and inside for six already. He's looking out the window, finding the farthest point he can. I follow his gaze through a yard, past a metal fence topped with razor wire, a concrete wall and then another concrete wall; the female prison next door. He looks back at me, eyes questioning. Looks right into me.

"Tell me this. Do you value your freedom?"

I smile ruefully. Or maybe it's just the nerves.

"I do since I've been working here, yes"

I don't add that I do since my partner was diagnosed with cancer as well.

Isla goes direct to her Mammy in the morning. She climbs over me as usual. But I get just a passing cuddle. She cosies up to her Mammy, kisses and strokes her. Wants to see the line that comes out her right breast, the dressing that holds it in place. Wants to see the wound that's healing on the other side where a breast once was. Anna pulls her vest top down one side after the other. Isla takes her Mammy's teddy, places it on the remaining breast.

237

"Does that feel better Mammy?"

Anna smiles, still has her eyes closed.

"Yes darling"

She'll be wondering about today's visit to hospital, if her immunity has risen enough for her to receive her third chemotherapy. If she can tick another one off, mark that halfway stage.

It hovers as still as it can in the gusting wind. Eyes trained for movement. Ready to dive any second. But it must have seen us out the corner of its eye; one man and his dog. And so it tips its wing and dips to the left, hitches a ride on an updraft. Round the corner of the island we go and there it is; above the cliff, still searching.

You can see it in her face these days. A gauntness. And her head's more pointed too. Or is that just my imagination? Regardless, it's in her eyes that the difference is most noticeable. They've lost their spark, are darker and duller. And the eyelids are drooping a little. Creasing the line that runs out from the bottom corner of her eyes deeper into her face. She sat down with a large plateful last night, knew it would be the last meal she'd be able to taste for more than a week. Then she fell asleep on the couch, was asleep before Joe. Could feel it taking effect, the combination of various drugs pumped slowly into her bloodstream. It's not supposed to have a serious effect for a couple of days. That's what they say. Anna wonders if it's psychological. You know it's coming so your body starts changing in expectation.

The sun appeared slowly over its liquid horizon. Just the top curve of a golden disc that threw laser beams across trembling ripples. I swam further from shore. Body, water, skin and bone lapping with early morning Mediterranean; sky, sea, myself as one. Nothing but blue water, blue sky and a golden seam that stitched us loosely together. Further up it came, this giant star of wonder from the centre of the solar system. Further up this giver of life and light, driver of climate, creator of energy. The sunshine illuminated my face and fed me. I turned over on my back, a playful porpoise. Pushed water with legs and cruised smoothly. Time wasn't chronological, wasn't structured. And it wasn't that it didn't matter but more that it didn't exist. I could vaguely remember the bar, the LSD tabs George bought us. Staring at a woman with a face like the moon. The DJ playing Lucy in the Sky with Diamonds as if he knew. Then classical music while some guy entranced us by waving fingers in front of our faces. I had images of fifty or sixty of us walking down the beach in the dark, myself and George laughing at everything and everyone. A bonfire and a wave of fuss and realisation that there wasn't one bottle opener between all of us. Bottles appearing from all directions. Passed from hand to hand as I shouted "bottle opener here – pass them along please." I opened them with my teeth, took a swig from each and passed them back. But all that was a dream that could have been days or months before. I looked around, spotted figures on the beach, the moon above them, still high in the sky, almost full and smiling. I could see its rays that softly pulled waves towards me, gently pulled waves inside me. And then a slim grey bird with orange beak, that skimmed the water and dipped its wing. Revelling in the thrill of natural freedom. And in its place, my new friend George, swimming his way towards me. Long curly hair billowing in the water around gentle eyes and face. I turned to the sun so we pointed the same way, dolphins about to play. But he hadn't come to swim. He'd come to mention something in his soft Irish lilt.

"Beautiful isn't it?"

I smiled. Words unnecessary. Insufficient.

We treaded water until some more words managed to appear from him.

"Aren't you supposed to be at work by now?"

I looked at my watch, still on my wrist, and it seemed he was speaking the truth. So I turned and swam back to shore, too peaceful to feel saddened by interruption. Wading back through the surf I realised I still had all my clothes on. Out the water I came, with a wave to those still on the beach. I took my boots off, poured sea out. Walked along the beach with them dangling in my hands. Past sun beds already put out by someone else. Up steps with watery footprints on concrete already warming. Past a sprinkling of early tourists, seawater dripping from my sodden clothes and body, from hair that slipped down my neck and shoulders. Up the path, boots still in hand, to the boss Nikos who looked at me part in pity, part in disgust, and threw his head back.

"You're sacked," he said. Then turned on his heels.

Billy Casper runs up those cobbled streets. He runs away from home, from family, from school with its bullying teachers and students. He runs away from the police, from society and all it preaches to him. He runs out of town and across the fields. Stands on a fence and looks up to the crumbling wall. Watches the kestrel spring from solid stone and soar into freedom. My students sit quietly through most of it. We've read the book and now we're doing the film. But now and then the odd comment is thrown in, an occasional remark of wonder met with murmurs of agreement. And when Billy starts training the kestrel, when he swings raw meat round and round in hoops and the kestrel sails through the air, thousands of years of evolution packed into muscle, bone and wing, into instinct and survival, I swear I can feel the atmosphere in the room deepen and heighten as men who have no freedom at all are reminded once again that the greatest things in life are the most simple and natural. And I daren't tell them I saw a kestrel yesterday morning whilst walking the dog, just minutes from my house.

Joe's naked, except for a pair of socks pulled up tight.

"I'm scared"

"Are you really scared?"

He often says he is when he wants a cuddle or conversation.

"Yes Daddy"

I take his hand, lead him back upstairs.

"Let's go and have a look"

We go up to his room. He climbs onto the windowsill and wraps himself in the curtain.

"Now, what can you hear?"

He listens while I cuddle him.

"Birds...shouting"

"Yeah. The birds love singing at sunset as well as sunrise don't they? Maybe they're singing each other goodnight songs. And do you know who that is shouting?"

"No"

I point to a garden on the right.

"See over there?"

"Yeah"

"Well there's a trampoline in that garden. And there must be bigger girls and boys living there because sometimes after you've gone to bed I can see them over the top of the fence jumping up and down and having fun. And one time they got a hosepipe and stuck it out the top window and blasted people with water in the garden below"

I tell him the dog barking is Niamh's dog, point out where she lives, next to Ester and Charlie. Mention how both our neighbours like to come and sit in their garden at night time, have a drink and chat. Then I point out a roof over on the right, say that could be Arthur and Eleanor's house. It's definitely their street.

"And Friday night's a happy night as well"

"How come?"

"Well, a lot of people work Monday to Friday so it's the start of the weekend now they're finished. And they won't have to get up for work in the morning so they're probably relaxing"

"Oh, like sitting on the couch eating crisps and watching telly?"

"Yeah, maybe having a little drink"

"A glass of white wine?"

"Yeah, or a beer maybe"

We listen another ten minutes or so. Then I put him to bed and kiss him goodnight, come downstairs after promising I'll ask his Mammy to go up for a cuddle.

Violence erupted in Malia almost every night. English men fighting with each other because they supported the wrong football team. Greeks responding to drunken provocation with violence. A Greek man was kicked to death. An Englishman stabbed to death the night later in retaliation. People I knew were arrested for dealing ecstasy and cannabis to tourists. Stalios and Rich sneaked me out food each day, even when I found a new job putting out sun beds every morning, putting them away every night. I phoned Anna but before I had the chance to tell her I'd been sacked she told me she was leaving her nursing course. Was coming to find me, wherever I was. I told her I hoped to be in Amsterdam in eight weeks time. Rich said we could get work there, unloading ships on the docks. My plan was to head via Eastern Europe, find work testing new drugs in Germany with an address I'd got from Ray who said he'd made a thousand pounds in two weeks. But within two weeks I'd been sacked again. There simply weren't enough tourists. The season was coming to an end. Thankfully I found a new job washing dishes ten hours a day, managed to save a couple of hundred pounds. Then one night I came back from work in the early hours of the morning to find my tent knifed into strips, my stuff raked through. So I spent the last few weeks revelling in the luxuriousness of a basic one room apartment. I'd just left it, was ambling across to work just a few days before I finally left when Marco came up to me, white as a sheet.

"What's wrong?"

"I've just seen my wife walking down the street," he said. "I don't know what to do"

I saw him the next day too. His wife had come to find him, take him back home after twelve long years. He clinched me in a bear grip and cried.

"And you know what? You'll never guess what? I'm a grandfather big feller. I'm a grandfather."

The day before I left I went to find him to say goodbye. His wife had gone back to Ireland to prepare for his homecoming. She'd bought him new clothes and he'd had a shave, was living in an apartment for the first time. Had to sleep with the door and window wide open because he was claustrophobic. He was taking his Yugoslavian mate Victor with him, was going to find him a good woman and a job.

Sleepy indifference spreads into sparkling smiles with the early morning news. Breakfast in the car because we're off to Harper Lees. We're driving just after seven and Isla asks if we're there yet before we've reached the end of our street. Three hours later we're all I Spy'd out and sick of looking for yellow and pink cars. But it doesn't matter because we're rumbling down the lane by the side of the river, rattling over cattle grids, in the heart of the Peak District. Past the sea monster, made from mine-shaft stone slabs, that swims in a sea of buttercups. Under a buzzard harassed by patrolling crows, by tape attached to posts that Isla says is a washing line for sheep to hang their socks on. Then we're hugging Building Granny and Grandad. And Joe and Isla are running with Stefan and Roland, children of Anna's soul sister Hester, while Anna picks salad and I sit on the wall, legs dangling, my back to the garden and the moose swing made of tyres. Looking out at sheep, hills, river and the cauliflower tree. I've been coming here seventeen years, ever since that stomach churning first drive down the lane to meet Anna's parents. It beckons Anna and her brother Richard and their childhood friends every year. Wild parties with sound systems have drifted into camping with children. Different herbs with the barbecue and bonfire. This is the place the Rolling Stones could have come to record one of their early albums, the perfect place to make music, create art or write. Children chatter. Shouts melt into the air when there's so much space around. I scan the pine forest, wonder how many kinds of life lie within. Then back to the big stone house behind, warming up for yet another welcoming weekend.

There's been a building here since 1252, built in the king's forest without the permission of Henry III himself, who journeyed up to Castleton to use the peak district for hunting. In 1968 a young couple called Gillie and Chris bought it, an empty shell last used for slaughtering pigs. The hooks they were hung up on are still inside the hall. And the stone slab they were butchered on is now beneath our feet when we sit on the outside bench.

Harper Lees is a place of refuge, of solace, of spiritual growth and balance. And it's my favourite place in the world. Those in need have been welcomed by Chris and Gillie for many years and still are. More cars arrive. Music plays out to the lucky few and to nonchalant sheep. Joe, Stefan, Roland and Izzy hide from adults, play adventures with sticks. Isla and Elysia play with dolls on the lawn. Richard and Louise prepare the food. Thomas toddles. Caffrey chews up tennis balls while Building Grandad has a smoke out the back with Peter, Hester, AJ and Rebecca. The barbecue is wafted. Pressures drift away with the smoke. And everything is balanced.

I'd just fallen asleep when the kicks came. Opened my eyes to German commands in police uniforms. Sleeping rough in a train station was not allowed. So out I went with all the other tramps, into a back alley where a knife was brandished and fighting began. I walked for hours in that cold October wind and rain. Tried to sleep behind a hedge but couldn't stop shaking. The address for the drug testing agency proved impossible to find and I'd ran out of money. Eventually I sneaked back into the train station where I met an East German Nazi skinhead who stole a car for the night and drove us out the city. We stopped in a lay-by, put the seats down, the warm air on. Spent the night there. In the morning he drove it back to the same place, left it for the owner. Unable to speak each other's language, but both without money and food, we simply hung out together for lack of anything else to do. And that's when Bodo walked up; a large and rather simple German man with a Dalmatian dog. And Bodo spoke reasonable English, which was welcoming. So despite my reservations about people scouring train stations for friends, I went with him and the skinhead to his flat for the night. The three of us watched telly and drank a bottle of clear spirits. Bodo assured me the pills he dropped into the bottle were simply "for flavouring." The next thing I knew he was pushing me, his dog licking my face. It was early morning. I'd fallen asleep on the floor.

"Come on," he said. "Let's go and get breakfast. I've sold my telly"

I lifted myself off the floor, looked around.

"Where's the other guy?"

"He's gone. It doesn't matter. Come on"

I realised my sleeping bag had gone too. Still, I hadn't eaten for two days so the promise of food was enough to get me out the house with anticipation. We came back fifteen minutes later with six bottles of extra strong beer.

"What about food?"

"Food? Hah! We don't need food. This is our breakfast"

After three each, he disappeared somewhere. I opened the kitchen cupboards, desperate for something to eat. For anything to eat. A slice of stale bread would have been heavenly. But there was nothing, not even a crumb. I even checked in the bin. And then, when he came back with four super strength beers from money he'd scrounged from a neighbour, I drank just one, wasn't interested in alcohol anymore. Bodo drank the other three and fell asleep. I waited until he was snoring, picked up my stuff and walked back out in the rain. Got kicked out the train station and walked for three hours to try and keep warm. I attempted to sleep in a disused building with my head between my knees but was too scared and too cold. In the morning I went to the post office to find fifty pounds sent by Anna. I'd asked for money to tide me over until I found the drugs testing place. So I said good riddance to Munich, got a train across country to Aachen, spent seven hours trying to get a lift and eventually hitchhiked to Amsterdam, desperate to find work and meet Anna in a week's time.

It sits on top of the cross, head twitching occasionally but body as still as if it were nailed there, smashed wine bottles on the concrete below. I walk past the church and wonder if it's the same kestrel I saw a few days ago.

A thirty-eight year old Glaswegian woman died of swine flu yesterday, the first in Britain. Her baby died this morning. The number of cases confirmed in Britain is now over one thousand, whilst unemployment has risen to 2.26 million. Question Time was full of anger towards politicians, for their expense claims and the recession. Meanwhile, Ronaldo signed for Real Madrid for eighty million pounds while eight Formula One teams are planning a breakaway championship because they don't agree with a forty million pound budget. And Susan Boyle is pulling out of the Britain's Got Talent tour through exhaustion. I pull into our drive, receive Isla's hugs around my legs. Anna tells me she had a lovely chat with the breast care nurse. Grants are available but she feels it's not right to take anything, that the money could be better spent elsewhere. The nurse tells her she's paid taxes every year. I tell her she's going down to half pay next month and we can hardly survive month to month anyway. She should accept whatever is offered. She had a chat about breast reconstruction as well, is still unsure. They've given her a DVD to watch.

Anna's back from seeing the geneticist at the Centre for Life. Her and her brother have to have colonoscopies when they're fifty-five. It searches for cancerous abnormalities in their large and small intestines. Isla has to have mammograms from the age of forty. They'd do them beforehand but exposure to radiation at an early age can be particularly damaging. So we need to be extremely vigilant until then.

She's stood in the kitchen with a hot water bottle wrapped in her dressing gown. A thermometer sticking out her mouth. I wondered why she'd made a funny noise when I spoke to her from the other room, so came to explore. She shakes with cold when I touch her hand, is worn down. Had to go straight into hospital when I got back from work. Needed to collect her sixth prescription of antibiotics. If her temperature goes up further she'll have go straight back in and stay the night, maybe longer. She's taking eight steroids every day during the week of chemotherapy now. They prevent unwanted reactions, lessen any side effects. But Anna feels they're making her touchy and aggressive, says she gets funny noises in her ears too.

She takes the thermometer out her mouth, holds it up, sighs.

"What? Is it alright?"

Nods.

"It's actually gone down, but just a little bit. By nought point one"

"Oh that's good"

"But if I start shaking in the middle of the night I have to go straight in. Okay?"

She gets up to go to the toilet. I lay there sleepy, realise she must be putting the kettle on, making drinks. She's still downstairs when Joe and Isla come in with a gift bag and two giant cards. That's when I remember its Father's Day. Joe gives me his card first, points his finger along it.

"That's Caffrey. That's me. That's Isla. That's you. And that's Mammy with a wig on. And that's a rainbow because look, it's sunny and it's raining"

And then it's Isla's turn. I can't work out who's who.

"It's me and you," she says. "You're the bald one in this picture Daddy. Mammy's not in it. And that's me with hair"

I suppose a phone box has some advantages over a train station. There's definitely not as much room for cold air to circulate. I'd walked around Amsterdam from ten p.m. until three a.m., looking for somewhere safe to put my head down. Never mind not allowing sleeping; the Dutch police wouldn't even allow me to sit down in the train station. For the first three nights I'd stayed at the Shelter, a strict Christian youth hostel in the middle of the red light district. It was the cheapest hostel in the city, situated there because that's where Jesus would have gone to save the souls of the devious, the disturbed and the otherwise damned. And there were plenty of those in Amsterdam. I'd got myself a work permit, spent half a day walking to the office and half a day walking back. Unfortunately I couldn't find any work and so ran out of money once more. I wandered around, no money for food or coffee shop. Was approached by drug dealers every five minutes. The next night I tried to sleep under some metal stairs in a building site, wishing I had my sleeping bag at the very least. After failing to sleep I walked to the train station, got thrown out by the police again, then went and stood in a phone box to get out the cold wind. The phone box next to me had three men inside smoking heroin. One of them came up to me so I let him in my phone box. He introduced himself as Marco from Genoa, gave me half his biscuit, half his packet of M&M's, said he was a heroin addict. He and his brother held up a post office with a gun and stolen car. His brother was shot dead by the police and he was taken out of prison after a month and placed in rehab. But he escaped and came to Amsterdam. He showed me the bullet wounds from his gun battle with the police, bought me two coffees from the Salvation Army. The police threw us out the phone box twice. We walked around in a circle and then went and laid down in the train station. He stopped someone stealing my bag and passport while I was sleeping. Then he slept and I stopped someone stealing what little change he had that had spilled out onto the floor.

I lay my books on the counter, walk past rows of chairs, take my seat behind a desk, already beginning to feel the heat. Then the library starts to fill and people take seats right at the front. They talk quietly to each other, don't look at me. And I don't know if they feel more vulnerable or I do. There's a fifteen minute wait while Lin runs back for a corkscrew. Warm buttered scones are handed round with cheese, a selection of nuts and nibbles, fruit juice and wine. The odd nervous smile comes my way and I think to myself; why did I agree to this? I'm not even sure what I'm supposed to be doing.

And then it starts. So I ask each in turn what they would like me to talk about and pray I'll be able to answer. Then I start talking. And somewhere along the line I get to that point where I notice the clock and think, "God, have I been rambling on that long?" And my inner voice is going "Look mate, people are doing their best to feign interest but they're just being polite. You know it, I know it, so let's not kid ourselves eh?" And I can't remember what the question was anyway. But I know I've been answering it, or not, for the past fifteen minutes at least. And then someone else asks me a question and it's a reprieve. I nod, saved for the moment. It's a question I'm interested in, reasonably knowledgeable about. So I take off in another direction. But after another few minutes of talking I realise I'm just throwing into the ring anything that vaguely resembles an answer. That I'm jumping all over the place in haphazard fashion, answering questions as soon as they're out of mouths instead of allowing five seconds for germination. I wonder if my face is going red. I know I'm sweating more than usual, that my glass of voice-saving water is very nearly finished. And when do these events finish? Because people keep nodding heads and I keep rambling. Someone leaves, says they're too hot. Two others leave without saying anything, walk out as I ramble on. And then somehow, but I'm not sure how, the whole thing comes to a finish and most people drift off. I have a chat with someone who's interesting and picks up on points. And I apologise and make excuses for not being structured and say I will be next time. But I forge a connection with her that's a welcoming relief from what went before. And we go into slight depth about something mentioned earlier and I start to gain confidence again. But then she has to leave so I say goodbye to the wonderful library staff and walk home, not knowing if I was a success, a partial success or a complete and utter failure. And then I get home and realise I shouldn't be so self-obsessed anyway.

The distance between central Amsterdam and Schipol Airport is nineteen kilometres. I know because I walked every one of them. When I saw Anna heading towards me I started to cry. But then she was with me, sunk into my arms, and nothing else mattered. We got the bus to town, booked into a cheap and seedy hostel so we could have our own room, four and a half months since we'd last seen each other. But after two nights of passion it was back to The Shelter. Male and female dormitories and a midnight curfew. We had no choice. Anna had two hundred pounds left of her bursary and I had nothing. And there was no sneaking into each other's dorms because staff came round with a torch at half past midnight checking you were in your own bed with the light off. We signed on at work agencies, visited them every morning without success. I walked to the docks but couldn't find work there either. Amsterdam was full of foreigners hoping to find work and live its coffee shop culture. The Shelter was no exception. But as time went by some started to get desperate. One lad decided he had no alternative than to become a rent boy. Others disappeared to God knows where. Soon, the only sustenance we could afford was a cone of chips with mayonnaise and a couple of smokes each day. Free hot chocolate and biscuits enticed us to daily bible class. But the only real salvation came from an ageing Geordie who'd gone to Amsterdam for a weekend twenty-three years before and never got round to returning. Him and an eccentric musician from New Zealand called Greg. The Geordie hadn't been able to afford hostels for years and consequently knew what to do when you were down and out or almost there. He gave us two scrumpled tickets for The Missionary, a free daily meal cooked by catholic nuns. We found it following the desperate down a back alley. At first we were hesitant. It looked like a dead end. But then we saw mingling in a doorway. Down we went, reassured, until we were stood in front of a nun about four feet tall looking up at us in judgement and pity. She took our tickets. Stared at us as if our souls weren't worth saving. Then stood aside and let us through. Into a large and shabby rectangular room we went, three parallel wooden tables running the whole length. A huge figure of a weeping Christ on the cross. I slipped my gold ring into my pocket and fifteen minutes later the place was full. We looked around at the assorted rabble of over one hundred, some of whom looked extremely dangerous and one, with a knife scar across his head, who was staring right at me. Still, the smell of warm food drifted across the worn table top and the impatient clink of cutlery grew louder and louder. And then the head nun, or whatever they're called, walked in and commanded silence. Ten long minutes of prayers pathetically mumbled by the starving and filthy followed, before bowls of stew with tiny slivers of meat were handed down tables. And all us grateful down and outs slopped it eagerly into greedy mouths.

The afternoon sun is in a scorching mood, burning the mist away without even trying. I watch a house martin dive from its nest above Isla's window, swoop across the road and up into the air, swing its body round and return. It looks such fun. It's not getting food, just flying for the thrill of it. I listen to its soft melodious chirp, wonder whereabouts in Africa it stayed for the winter. And I marvel how it can fly such a distance feeding along the way. How it chose to build a nest right above my little daughter's bedroom window. Then I'm walking down the path at the bottom of our road, and it's quieter than usual down the dene. Just the occasional twitter, the odd coo of a wood pigeon. They must all be conserving energy in the stupefying heat. A heron lifts off without sound, floats effortlessly away. I see its mate, feet dunked in a pond left by the flooding spring tide. Their heads don't turn as Caffrey and I approach but they're keeping an eye on us. And then the first one floats off again, another fifty metres further down. The remaining one waits a few moments, then takes off lower, smoother, like an arrow. We circle them over dry grass, one with a long thin neck straight up, the other curled like a hook. We look down at what little water is left by the retreating tide. Notice plants that grow on the bed floating on top, shimmering silver in the sunlight. Glittering leaves that turn green further up in the shade, strewn over treacherous stepping stones. The cattle have come down to the water's edge to cool off. Two calves are busy licking each other. A bull in the water up to his knees rolls his eye at me. Lifts a hoof out of sticky mud.

We watch the DVD as soon as the kids are in bed, a welcome respite from the radio continuously telling us about the death of Michael Jackson. But if I'm expecting some News of the World before and after boob job then I'm in for a reality shock. There are three types of breast reconstruction. The lattissimus dorsi flap. The abdominal muscle flap (commonly known as a tram flap). And the synthetic breast implant. They all require general anaesthetic and a breathing tube. For the lattissimus dorsi the surgeon cuts out a section of tissue and skin from the back and folds it round to the front to form the new breast. For a tram flap the surgeon opens up an incision in the chest and then uses fat and muscle from the abdominal wall, or if there's not enough tissue, from the lower back. He slides this tissue beneath the skin to the mastectomy site to form a breast mound. Great care is taken to preserve the blood supply it says. And finally, the synthetic breast implant. The surgeon opens up an incision at the mastectomy site and inserts a balloon-like tissue expander. Over a period of weeks salt water is regularly injected into the tissue and expander. Then the expander is taken out and a permanent synthetic implant is inserted. Decisions can then be taken on whether or not a nipple and areola reconstruction is wanted and if so these are done separately, using tissue from the inner thigh or ear. The breast reconstruction means hospitalisation for three to five days, presumably five with bouncing young children at home. And the recovery period is three to six weeks before any further nipple and areola surgery can be considered. And even though the DVD uses computerised 3D models it immediately becomes apparent that these operations are much more serious and dangerous than the removal of the breast in the first place. I try not to imagine Anna being cut in any of these ways. My naive and stupid thoughts of her having a nice new pair of breasts are brought crashing down. I've changed my mind. I don't want her to go through all this. But Anna's erring on the side of reconstruction.

"I want to be able to go swimming with the kids again," she says. "I want to be able to wear a bikini without people staring at me, feeling sorry for me"

PART VIII

The area has a beauty to it, of that there can be no doubt. Old town houses, small curved bridges. Lights that reflect off canals, spread across water like brush strokes from famous Dutch masters. And then there's the windows; girls brazen in underwear and lingerie. Girls of every colour and origin to choose from. Sometimes a slightly older woman with a stern look and a whip. On occasions a woman with extra folds of flesh, one for the fetishists and the drunken stags to point and laugh at. Mannequins of real flesh in window after window. They move around and tempt you, stretch arms up behind heads, straighten hair, dance their little dance. Swing knicker elastic. They'll close the curtains, peel their underwear off, let you come inside. Most of the time, I couldn't look them in the eye.

Greg led the way, guitar tucked under arm, looking more like some children's TV presenter than a rock 'n' roller. He stopped by a bridge, put his guitar down, fastened his coat.

"Here will do"

I rubbed my hands together, looked around. The woman in the nearest window looked bored. I watched her get up, go over to the sink, pick something up then sit on her bed again. She sat behind glass in knickers and bra, painted her nails.

"It's not very busy"

"It's November," said Greg. "And it's freezing and raining. If it was summer this street would be mobbed"

"Just our luck," said Anna, offering me a plastic cup.

I took it and shook.

"It doesn't sound very good this"

Shook again.

"In fact, it doesn't sound at all"

Anna took some small change out, added it to both our plastic cups so they rattled.

And then Greg picked up his guitar and started to play.

Unfortunately myself and Anna didn't know many songs, were too stoned to remember anyway. Greg tried a few Beatles numbers but we kept forgetting the words. He wanted us to sing, shake cups and approach people, thought it would get us more money. After a couple of embarrassing attempts, he put his guitar down and pondered. Then he looked up and smiled, taught us the words to 'Do Your Ears Hang Low? Do They Swing To and Fro?' Made us do the actions. Seconds later, someone walked past, smiled and gave some change. We increased our repertoire to three, adding 'She'll Be Coming Round The Mountains' and 'How Much Is That Doggy in the Window?' The actions made us a little warmer. People dropped loose change into our plastic cups, pennies to them but little parcels from heaven to us. And we had fun, lots of it. Maybe most of the people who walked past were stoned or drunk. Perhaps they pitied us. But we made twenty-one guilders that first night. It wasn't enough to pay for beds at the hostel but it was enough for food and smoke.

And so we went out earlier the next night, hoping to make more. But it was quieter and colder. We only made twelve guilders but the girl in the nearest window recognised us. Stopped painting her nails and danced to the music. And for a few moments, everything was in sync. But she was busier than we were. We leant on railings and timed men, watched them hurry away after. Fifteen minutes seemed about normal. And then the woman opened her curtains and smiled at us.

I check Amazon, delight at how my book has soared through the rankings to 66,796. Take Joe to the leisure pool so he can climb onto the pirate ship, fire water cannons at my head. We play power rangers, jump the waves. After dinner I take him and Isla to the school playground to ride bikes and play on the obstacle course. We have a great time, but when we come back Anna responds to enthusiastic exclamations in an unusual subdued manner. When we have a moment to ourselves I ask her what's wrong.

"I'm sorry," she says, unable to hold my eye for more than a second. "I feel like I've missed out. And I feel guilty for not being there"

"It's only been a couple of hours," I tell her. "They've had a great time. And they were really happy to come home and see you"

"It's not just today," she says. "It's the last few weeks. I haven't been the same with them. I've been tired and run down. Or snappy and bad tempered"

I smile.

"So you've been a bit more like me then?"

But she's not in the mood for bad jokes so I try another tactic.

"We met eighteen years ago girl. Eighteen years. Our son is nearly six years old"

That makes her smile.

"It's amazing isn't it? How time whizzes by so fast? There's only six weeks left of your chemotherapy. And that's the main part over isn't it?"

She shrugs.

"I guess so"

And then she walks out the kitchen to find out what the children are doing.

Joe's still asleep when I leave the house for work. I kiss his forehead, whisper happy birthday. Tell Anna I want him to open his presents before I get back. It's not fair having to wait three extra hours. I kiss Anna goodbye, Isla too. She's delighted with herself because she's worn a nightie for the first time ever, wants to keep showing me it. The drive to work tells me three hundred and thirty-nine people in Britain have Mexican swine flu, confusing because I was told last week it was over a thousand. The Independent on

Sunday a few days ago wrote that the true extent of the outbreak is near to thirty thousand. Then the radio tells me a plane has disappeared off the radar after leaving Brazil for France. And it tells me a couple jumped to their death from Beachy Head cliffs with a dead child in a rucksack. At work I cover for an English Language teacher but all students except one want to talk about court claims and who's going to win the Premiership. I come home to Joe's birthday tea but all's far from happy. His friend Arthur's crying because of toothache. Isla's being unkind to Eleanor and Anna can't get Joe's second hand Playstation working. And being a technological dunce, neither can I. So I take Isla upstairs but she's past it and refuses to brush her teeth. I get angry, throw the duvet over her. She swings her legs and kicks me in the face.

I watched them; those advert teeth and genuine smiles. That pleated skirt as she walked. Clean and fresh. The antithesis of me. I watched them when we were invited into the back room for bible class. They didn't frown at the state of my dirty jeans, at the mark they may have made on their comfy pale sofa. They looked me in the eyes when they gave me coffee and biscuits, always asked our point of view when they discussed the day's topic. They wanted to help, of that I was certain. They wanted to help and believed they could. Believed without any doubt whatsoever that I only had to do one thing, that all of us invited into the back room only had to do one thing. And then all our troubles and worries would be over. And I wanted that to happen so much. I was fed up walking round Amsterdam's work agencies every morning to hear the same answer time and time again. Depression hung its heavy cloak around me more and more and I was becoming too tired to shrug it off. Perhaps if I could have cuddled up to Anna at night, I would have felt different. But I had accepted her into my life of adventure and provided her with nothing. Not even a comforting arm at night time. A telephone call home found my Mam in ill health. Images of all those people I'd met on my travels flashed like visions; people like me, searching for something extra from life. The cynical side of me scoffed at that pleated skirt, those pump shoes and tights, the cardigan with childish pattern. But my position was hardly one to assume arrogance from. And anyway, they had an answer primed and ready; a Dutch skinhead covered in tattoos who'd been imprisoned for murder. He'd found the right way, had been cynical too beforehand. He'd scoffed and sinned and enjoyed them both. But deep inside he knew there was something else, that there had to be something else. And since he'd found the truth his life had been transformed. I stayed behind after bible class one afternoon, asked for a one-to-one. Of course they would oblige. It was their life's mission, to save people like me. And here they had someone perfectly ripe for conversion. I walked down the docks with Anna, talked about religion and what difference it might make to our lives. Anna was respectful and interested as always, but not sure that was her path. We stopped for a shared cone of chips on the way back, bumped into Tom and Timbere in Dam Square, a charming pair of best friends from Middlesbrough and Rio de Janeiro. They invited us to a coffee shop. But I had more important things to consider than getting stoned again.

Do I look at women's breasts more these days? I ponder this question after peeling my eyes away from a pair in front of me. She was about to look up and I didn't want to get caught. I nod a few trivialities instead and wonder. And then, when her eyes return to the credit card payment in front of her, my eyes return once more to her breasts. Like most men, I appreciate the beauty as much as the practicality. The soft inviting curves and tender flesh. But I also remember Joe clamped on for all he was worth, tiny hand gripping her waist, eyes wide open. Sucking as much milk as he could possibly get as often as he possibly could. I receive my credit card back and say goodbye to the eyes, confident I haven't been spotted. Then I walk outside and wonder; do most women take their breasts for granted? Are they proud of them? Do they realise how lucky they are to still have two? Or have they been sucked into the media world of models, of certain size, of sexuality and perfect symmetry?

The heron stands still as a statue, waits patiently a hundred metres from the early morning tide. We have the beach to ourselves and there is much to have, its pale soft folds filling much of the view, any noise the rippling tide may make too far away to register. Two hundred years ago this beach had over seven thousand men on it, and all for the love of one woman. The Duke of York, Commander in Chief of the British Army, was in love with Lord Delaval's daughter. And so, in a bid to impress her, he brought his army north for manoeuvres. Paraded and inspected them on the beach under her gaze.

She turned him down.

It's everywhere we turn. Newspaper, radio and television. It's the topic of conversation in the staffroom, the butt of many jokes. And of course it means nothing unless you have a personal connection. It's just another story, like BSE and bird flu. But this is something that's deadly dangerous to Anna, that's growing, getting nearer and nearer. The irony wouldn't contain even trace amounts of humour; survived cancer and killed by flu. A man I met on the poetry scene has just recovered from cancer. He and his wife became paranoid and introverted. Went supermarket shopping at night time when there was hardly anyone about. Wouldn't accept flowers as gifts in case of infection. He's older and therefore, I presume, more vulnerable. But we can begin to understand now. It's out there, invisible. Hiding on door handles. Propelled at six hundred miles per hour from people's noses and mouths.

Kathy smiled as she beckoned me into the back room. We moved past the comfy sofa towards the far corner, where two chairs faced each other, a round wooden table in between. She moved her wavy black hair behind her ear, put her hands underneath her chin and asked what was on my mind. I told her I was depressed at constantly looking for work but never finding any. I told her I was fed up being hungry all the time, worrying about having a place to put my head down. I told her about sleeping rough in

Egypt, Munich and Amsterdam. I told her my Mam was unwell, how I worried about her. I told her my Daddy died two weeks before my second birthday, that my Mam had married again, that I had two fathers, one in this world and one somewhere else. I told her I loved Anna dearly but that since she'd left nursing training nothing had gone right for us and it filled me with guilt. And I told her I desperately hoped there was something more to life than that which I had found so far. That yes, it felt like there was something missing. Kathy took my hand and smiled. Let Jesus into your life she said. Let Jesus into your life and you will never look back. Your worries will dissolve and in the afterlife you will rise to heaven with angels. I wiped away tears and asked about my family. Would they rise to heaven as well? Yes she said; if they take Jesus into their lives too. If they see the light shining from you and follow your lead. If they pray every day to the one true God.

"But what about my Daddy?" I asked. "He's already dead. Will he be waiting in heaven for me?"

She paused for the first time, uncertain.

"Did he pray every day?"

"No," I said. "Or at least I don't think so. But he was a good man, a kind and generous man. And he did believe in God. He just didn't pray every day to him"

Another pause.

"Will he be waiting in heaven for me?"

Her eyes lowered then came back up again.

"No," she said. "God only allows those who pray daily into his pearly gates. And if he didn't pray every day then he won't be in heaven"

Anna asks for the second or third time if her hair is growing back. Here we go again I think, as she lowers her head and places it near my face.

"It looks the same as ever"

"Does it?"

"Yeah...ah hang on, wait there"

I pull her head closer, inspect further. She'd never been completely bald close up, still had tiny dead hairs rooted in and refusing to fall out. But these ones look soft, like they might be fresh and new.

"I think it is growing back"

"Really?"

"Yeah"

I never thought there was a chance they would grow back before her chemo finished.

"They're a funny colour though"

"Are they?"

I put my fingers to her head, look all serious.

"What colour are they then?"

"More like a reddish ginger colour"

"Are they?"

"Mmmm...or maybe grey actually"

She pulls her head round to face me, studies me. My smile gives her the answer.

"Is it really growing back?"

I rub her head a couple of seconds with the flat of my palm.

"Yes, it really is darling"

And so she walks away with a curious smile on her face. Off to find a mirror and twist her head.

I knew what I had to do as soon as I came off the phone. Anna was outside the booth, watching the world go by, or at least Amsterdam's section of it. I didn't tell her at first. I couldn't. She'd left nursing college, a whole career and way of life, to come to Amsterdam and be with me. I just linked her arm and walked away, down the road as the rain grew heavier. Anna said nothing. She'd seen my face, knew it was serious. By the time we got halfway down the road the rain was coming down in torrents and the odd crack of lightning split open the black sky as if God himself was angry with my decision to snub him.

I pulled Anna into a doorway, grabbed hold of her, hugged tight. She lifted her head out my chest, looked up, saw tears streaming down, guilt ridden eyes.

"What is it?"

"I have to go home"

She looked puzzled.

"It's my Mam. She's not well"

Anna nodded, understood. She knew a son must return home if he feared his mother may be about to die.

We hugged some more, and then more again. Our tears poured out with the rain. Then we went to find a coffee shop.

Radio 4 tells me unemployment is swelling, with twenty-three thousand people being made redundant every week. I arrive back from work and study Anna's head. It's tufty, wispy. Sticking up like hair on a new-born baby that's been bathed for the first time. But her eyelashes and eyebrows have nearly all gone. I realise now how they symbolise femininity much more than hair. With hair it could be a choice, a fashion statement. You don't look like a victim when your hair's gone. Not like you do when you have no eyebrows and eyelashes. Now there's just pencil to mark where hair once was above her eyes. And she has to wear glasses much more because her eyelashes aren't there for protection.

She's slumped on the couch, trying to keep her eyes open, can only manage it for two seconds at a time. Dilated pupils blurring and frosting with chemotherapy drugs that patrol her every cell, search for skulking tumours. Behind us the conservatory roof hammers with the noise of pouring rain, as it did all night. I pop my head through the living room door, watch water dripping through in four different places, dropping into Tupperware's with constant little splashes.

"I must get that roof fixed"

When I turn back round Anna's giving me a look that's managed to bore its way through all those drugs. I've been saying I should get the roof fixed for months but only remember when it's raining. And it needs to be dry for me to do something about it.

She pulls herself up straighter.

"One of Claire's kids might have swine flu," she says. Claire is our child-minder. Joe and Isla go there three times a week after school.

I smile stupidly. Don't know what to say.

"One lad's Mam has it too, a lad in Isla's class. Helen told me. They'll be cooped up next to each other in this rain"

A deepening sense of foreboding starts to envelop us both. Not that Isla cares. Her main ambition today is to be able to hop. She comes into the living room in a determined manner but falls straight over.

"I'm thinking about taking them out of school," says Anna. "There's only one week left 'til the summer holidays start. It will be more difficult for me to catch it then"

"I'll see if I can take time off," I say. "I'm sure my boss will let me"

Isla hops through, manages five or six, seems really pleased with herself. Then looks into the garden and sings out of tune.

"It's raining, it's pouring, the snowman is boring"

"But then I think it's just me," says Anna, "being really paranoid. We can't keep them away from Arthur and Eleanor, their other friends. Helen works in a pharmacist five days a week. What if she gets it? What if they get it? Their lives need to be as normal as possible. It's not fair to isolate them because of something that might happen to me"

Carole comes to the door to drop Molly off. She takes a tissue from her pocket and blows her nose. I say thanks and shut the door on her quickly. Walk back into the living room.

Where Anna pleads through dilated eyes of paranoia.

"It said on the radio its spreading much more swiftly than they ever imagined. 0.5 per cent of people who get it will die. That's one in every two hundred"

I walk forwards and sit next to her, pull her into me and kiss her head through the scarf. More danger signs stroll through my mind, like they know there's nothing I can do about them. You can ask six year olds and three year olds to wash their hands a million times but you can't supervise them every time. And that's just your own kids. I work in a prison where nine hundred men are kept in tiny confined spaces and over a thousand staff are employed. Swine flu would wreak havoc there.

"And what if I do get it?" she continues. "Or if I get a cold and I'm worried it might be swine flu? They're not going to let me into hospital to get checked out are they? Where loads of vulnerable and ill people are, who might catch it off me? And even if they have to, they'll try and delay things as much as they can. And what will the impact be on me?"

We sit on the couch and say nothing until Anna finishes the topic once and for all.

"I know I'm going to get it," she says. "I know I am"

Each night the queue got longer, though it was more of a stoned gathering than anything resembling orderly. And then someone looked at a watch and raised eyebrows.

"Twelve o'clock. Time to go in"

Nervous shuffling. Much looking at feet. Nobody wanting to be the first. But eventually, as always in life, someone had to be the bravest. And so in we went, like a drunken snake that part weaved part staggered through the door and past the desk. Past Kathy with the pleated skirt who cast pitying eyes on those who had sinned once more. Anna had more reason than most to toe the line, to worry about such judgement. She'd put her name on the cleaning list. Success didn't provide a wage but it did mean free board, and so competition was understandably fierce and quite desperate. Anna put her best argument forward though, and perhaps staff saw a forthcoming split as an opportunity worth pursuing. A cleaning job meant partial integration into the world of staff. If they couldn't persuade me then perhaps they could tempt Anna. And with Anna's head turned to salvation, the biblical net would surely fall on me too. She got the job, was due to start the day I left.

I said goodbye to Kathy. Both my mother and I would be added to the daily prayer list she said. Then further goodbyes to the many friends we'd made, who all promised to look after Anna. Don't worry I said, I'll be back in a couple of weeks. And then back to that seedy hostel again, for a final night. We had a couple of drinks downstairs, noticed two members of Shelter staff hiding in a dark corner with a joint and a beer. Then upstairs to a smoke and a game of strip poker. And what was destined to be my last ever night in Amsterdam.

Isla's awake but hasn't moved from her bed or spoken. Usually she comes into our room, climbs in our bed as soon as she's woken up. Groans if we send her back because it's too early. Not this time. I pop my head around the corner of the door frame and there she is. Eyes wide open, lying still and peaceful. Just the offering of a cursory glance towards me this morning. She's listening to the baby house martins chirp chirping in their little nest right above her bedroom window.

Anna unfolds the Observer, spreads it out in front of her. She doesn't normally read the paper on a Sunday morning. Usually wants breakfast finished, teeth brushed, the family out for a walk with Caffrey whatever the weather. But she hasn't got the energy today. She's going back for a lie down in half an hour. I ask the kids if they want to stroke Mammy's head, feel her hair growing back again. They queue up, take it in turns. Isla grins. Joe cheers, strokes it a second time.

"It's all soft," he says.

Anna smiles, reads the front page awhile, decides she's had enough, hands it back to me.

"They're talking about opening temporary mortuaries," she says. "Shorter funerals"

I'm on the Playstation with Joe when the phone rings. Anna answers it quickly. She's worried about Louise, her brother's wife. She was round there earlier, checking out the baby room when I called her. It's beautiful she said. You should see it. It's beautiful. But Louise had to go into hospital because she couldn't feel the baby move. And she hadn't phoned Anna back as requested. Don't worry I said. There's only a week to the due date. There isn't any room to move. She'll be fine. Three words tell me this isn't true. I watch Anna as she puts her hand to her mouth. Just three words but they stretch to breaking point when they come out:

"I'm so sorry"

She says it again and again. It's all she can say.

I tell Joe it's time to stop the Playstation. He pleads but I insist. I take him upstairs and ask him to choose a book. Then, when he realises I'm not actually reading it to him, he curls up in a ball and groans. I leave him there, go back downstairs. Anna's in the back garden shaking, tears streaming down cheeks. I hold her tight. There's nothing I can say. She goes inside to write a letter to Louise and Richard. I start tidying the kitchen. After half an hour Joe comes down and Anna tells him his baby cousin is dead. He looks up at her face with a puzzled expression.

"Why?"

Anna leans down, strokes his hair.

"It just happens sometimes darling. It's very rare but sometimes it just happens"

He groans.

"But I was looking forward to having another cousin to play with"

274

"I know sweetheart"

"Did it get ran over?"

"No, it just stopped breathing. It was still inside Louise's tummy"

"Is Aunty Louise dead as well?"

"No, she's not. Just the baby"

They walk back upstairs, hand in hand. After five minutes I go to the bottom of the stairs and listen.

"Can you tell Daddy to save the Lego Star Wars game. I don't want to do level one again, no way"

It's what he knows, what he understands. I hear nothing else. I guess she's holding him tight.

I walk Caffrey, post Anna's letter. The sun's going down, orange turning over to dark blue. We're only out fifteen minutes. Caffrey runs up to the front door. I look up, attracted by the noise. Isla's sleeping safely in her bed and the house martins are tucked up in their nest above her, chirping away like excited children in a tent. Anna's having a glass of wine outside in the dark. I join her. We sit in silence and then she finishes first and goes to bed. I finish my wine, listen to the breeze blowing against cauliflowers and broccoli that have been battered by wind and rain, sent to seed. And I think to myself; don't ever say that things were meant to be, that everything is meant for a reason.

Each night, as the sun went down, wolves could be heard howling from all directions. We put our heads on pillows, closed our eyes to their haunting call. There was a reassuring presence in their long plaintive cries second time around, as if they'd moved nearer to welcome us home, to the place we loved more than anywhere else. The place we fell in love. No more walking the streets getting hassled by dealers, rejected by work agencies. No more worrying where the next meal would come from. Anna flew back to England. We spent time in London, a wonderful Christmas with my parents, New Year with Anna's family. Then back to Israel and Afiq, the start of our adventures and romance. The place our hearts always remained. Anna worked in the gardens with Marla. I took hand saws and clippers, pruned trees in the avocado orchards. Drove tractors with my t-shirt wrapped around my head. Tom, who we'd met in Amsterdam, followed Anna and I out to Afiq and worked in the avocadoes too. He was twenty years older than me, had left Middlesbrough after a painful divorce. We worked hard, then relaxed in the shed and played poker for a couple of hours. After work, we walked through valleys most days, just Anna and I usually. We spotted the usual; eagles, vultures and hawks, coyote, deer and wolves. We passed a family of tortoise out for a mid afternoon stroll, warmed ourselves with rock rabbits at sunset. Disturbed by a very close rustling one afternoon, we stood and watched as a Giant Syrian Mongoose came out the bush, looked at us in astonishment for a full ten seconds, then walked away nonchalantly, swinging its bum. And then, down our Kinneret Valley towards our Sea of Galilee and its sparkling surface, we picked wild flowers, olives and almonds from the trees that flourished below bombed out Syrian houses.

Anna walks with her arms folded, while the children run ahead laughing and jumping in muddy puddles. Sophie Elizabeth Peace was born today, weighing six pounds and two ounces. The cord was wrapped around her neck three times but lots of babies are born okay that way. It will go down as unexplained, like about half of all babies dying in the womb just before birth. She's staying with her Mummy and Daddy in hospital for a few days so they can have some time together as a family.

Down the edge of the valley we went, sliding on bums. The soles of our shoes creating clouds of dust around our heads, dislodging rocks that hurtled far below. At first we kept the ladder with us, bringing it down little by little. Then we pushed it like a sledge, watched it slide in front. The larger rocks were left untouched. Recently discovered diamond backed snakes ensured that. Across the valley the other side loomed, far steeper and more dangerous. We'd climbed halfway up that side earlier in the day, had disturbed an eagle just a few yards away. It flew out with huge wings, eyeballed us back on the cliff face. We decided climbing near nests was a stupid idea, clambered straight back down. Then, walking along the valley floor, still astonished at the sight of an eagle so close, we discovered the hole, or to be more precise, nearly fell down into it. It must have been fifteen feet deep and ten feet wide. And there was something at the bottom, down in the darkness of the shade. So back to the kibbutz we went, to borrow a ladder. And then down the edge we scrambled; two men from Teesside and a girl from the Peak District. While everyone else we knew in England was working nine to five, immersing themselves in the wearying daily grind of life, we were spending the whole afternoon exploring a hole in the middle of the Golan Heights. Unfortunately, when we got there the ladder wasn't long enough. Tom kept hold of my legs as I lay down then lowered and dropped it into the hole. It reached four or five feet from the top. Then Tom lowered himself down to the top rung, climbed down and held the bottom whilst I followed. Anna stayed where she was, peered down as we raked around. There were bones, in the shadowy corner. But we couldn't work out if they were human or animal.

She's lying in her moses basket. Pink hat pulled down over forehead, blanket pulled up over jumpsuit. Her tiny fingers curl round mine as if she were still breathing. Anna didn't want to let go of her, kissed her head over and over, wanted desperately to pick her up and cuddle her. Eventually she stood aside to let others get closer.

Sophie Elizabeth Peace...

She's a beautiful baby, tall and elegant. And she would have had a beautiful and lucky life to live, with a loving family

278

on both sides, an adoring Mummy and Daddy. She would have grown up to be caring and loyal like her parents, to be curious and understanding rather than jump with two feet into judgement. She would have grown up to be one of the finest of this world; no doubt would have dedicated her life to helping others less fortunate than herself, like so many in her family. But that opportunity has been taken away from her. And so she'll always be loved for what she is; a beautiful baby girl with long fingers and a button nose.

Both her grandparents are present as well as her Uncle Richard and Aunty Anna. The chaplain baptises her with water Anna brought for herself in case she felt choked up. Building Grandad points out how wonderful and appropriate it is that a female has baptised his granddaughter. Sophie's parents are dignified and remarkable given the circumstances. Richard still manages to crack jokes that make everyone laugh. Then the chaplain leaves and Building Granny smiles underneath tears.

"All she's known has been peace"

Her Mummy smiles.

"And comfort," says Anna. "And warmth"

I could tell Anna had been up to something as soon as she came into our apartment. "Close your eyes," she said, hands rooted behind her back.

I did as I was told.

"Put your hands out"

I offered them gingerly, unsure what to expect.

"Happy birthday darling"

My fingers rustled and crackled. And I opened my eyes to a large packet of Draculina; my favourite Greek crisps.

She smiled. This was a sacrifice, a gesture of love. For the last two days we'd eaten nothing but sugar sandwiches. It was all we could afford. Our money was almost out and neither of us had managed to find a job since arriving back in Malia. If we didn't find anything within two days we'd be penniless and homeless.

"Anna. You shouldn't have"

She looked apologetic.

"It's your birthday. I had to get you something"

I ripped the bag open, offered it to her.

She refused, insisted, said it was my birthday. I should have them all to myself.

And so I scoffed them one after the other as she watched me.

Half an hour later Tom knocked on the door. He'd found something, wanted me to follow. It really was turning into a birthday to remember. Through the quiet streets of Malia we went, the influx of tourists not yet descended, past the place where Anna found a job but got sacked three hours later for refusing to belly dance on the bar. Down to the beach and the secret horde.

In a few weeks the sand would burn delicate English soles. Would host fumbling and fucking couples in the darkness. Tom stopped at the bottom of a beach bar, looked around to see if we were alone. The sun moved slowly downwards, hadn't yet drawn all the light away. Then, when he was certain there was no one else present, he moved towards a pile of bin bags. I followed him up, stepped off the beach, watched him rip one open with fingernails.

"Shit"

He wiped hands on jeans, started on another.

"This feels more like it"

Held one aloft and beamed proudly.

"Is that a doughnut?" I asked.

"Course it is mate. There's loads of them. There was last night as well but I found them too late to come and get you"

He stuffed one in his mouth, opened the bag further. There must have been two dozen in there. We gorged ourselves on four or five each. Custard doughnuts. Jam doughnuts. Chocolate coated doughnuts. And then Tom took his t-shirt off and wrapped a dozen up. And we left the beach, where Tom put his head down every night. And we walked back up the streets of Malia, proud hunter gatherers. Took our findings to Anna, waiting eagerly in the apartment we were about to lose.

I drive to work listening to Radio 4 tell of a Sudanese woman arrested for wearing trousers, deemed indecent clothing. She's likely to face forty lashes and an indefinite fine. But she won't take them off, is prepared to face the consequences. Over the Tyne I go, beckoned by a flaming sunrise invaded by tower blocks and factory smoke. Stood higher than this, surveying it all and the hills beyond; the Angel of the North, iron clad steel arms still not tired after all these years. I press play on the CD player; Jonny Cash live at San Quentin Prison. He sings Darling Companion with June Carter Cash, then I Don't Know Where I'm Bound, written by a prisoner who's present. I think of prisoners where I work, wonder what will happen to them when they eventually get out. Then Jonny plays a new song he wrote especially for the concert, entitled San Quentin. The prisoners cheer wildly as he slates the prison system for being ineffective. And as I drive along these dales of Durham I can feel the energy and power from a concert that happened forty years ago on the other side of the Atlantic. My eyes start filling with tears. I even start to sob like a baby. I understand prison is needed, I'm not stupid. But I do see another side to prisoners, focusing as creative writing often does on elements of their thoughts and lives that don't include crime. I read their stories of better times, help with poems about cot deaths, take prisoners on time-lines. Travel with them to blues nights, to childhood and the queen's jubilee. To the first realisation that being black was not being part of things. I wipe tears away with the flat of my hand. Maybe emotions from recent events have been building inside without my knowledge. Anna had her last chemo yesterday. And it's Sophie's funeral tomorrow.

I sat on the wall, scanned tourists starting to wander down the main road. Seven planes had arrived in the last twenty-four hours. This was the start of it. The tourist season in full swing. With these people came our hopes, not just for survival but also for flourishing. And then I saw them, in their pale blue shirts. Off the wall I jumped, conscious of being too conspicuous but more concerned I get to Anna in time. I jogged past lazy tourists with the odd sidestep, the odd 'excuse me', found Anna on her usual corner. A couple had stopped, seemed interested, but this was no time for smiling pleasantries.

"The police are coming darling. We've got to go - quick"

She muttered apologies to the bemused couple, picked up the cardboard display and off we went, down a side street. Didn't bother to notify Tom keeping watch further down. Round the back of some apartments, dumped our stuff on the floor, not daring to spy back round the corner in case we got spotted. We stayed there fifteen minutes, hoped the Germans further down the road were spotted, had their wares confiscated. Theirs was a professional set up compared to ours. They had suitcases, a folding table. They had variety. And most importantly, they knew what they were doing and were good at it. We'd positioned ourselves further up the road to try and catch tourists before they saw how good they were. And we undercut them by half. I looked down at our cardboard display. We'd spent our very last money on six different coloured threads and some beads. Had practiced making friendship bands and hair wraps for two days nonstop. The first few friendship bands were awful but by the end of the first day we'd got the hang of it. Hair wraps were trickier. You needed the victim in front of you. The first few came back, complained they were falling out. We apologised and fixed them for free.

And we were just getting the hang of it when the police caught Anna whilst Tom and I were out looking for work. If they found her trading illegally once more they were going to put her in prison.

When we felt certain the police had gone, we returned cautiously to the main street. By eight p.m. Anna had been there ten hours, had made enough for two more nights at our room. We wandered back up to the old town, left Tom enjoying a free beer with a new found friend. Thought maybe we'd set up again around ten or eleven when people had eaten, had bought a few drinks. But the old Greek woman who owned the apartment was waiting for us at the door, wrinkled hands on wide hips.

"You have friend sleep"

"What?"

"You." She pointed accusingly at me. "You have friend sleep here"

I shook my head. "No – none of our friends have slept here"

"You must go"

Anna tried to reason. It wasn't true. Nobody had slept over, not even Tom, who recognised our need for privacy, said he was fine sleeping on the beach.

But the old woman wasn't interested in truth. And she wasn't interested in negotiation. She was interested in money.

"Please. You go now. I don't want police"

And so we packed our rucksacks and picked up our cardboard display. And left. The tourists had arrived. Things had changed. Some would have booked flights only, would need accommodation. Others would get thrown out of hotels. She could charge four times more than we were paying and that was all that mattered. A wander around the old town offered no reprieve. There were only a couple of vacant apartments and their owners weren't interested in workers either. Charges had shot up overnight. We didn't want to sleep with Tom, for as much as we loved him we were desperate to have as much time together as possible. And so, after failing to find any disused or empty buildings, we climbed stone steps on the side of an apartment and reached a concrete roof. Alone, apart from a washing line that stretched from one side to the other, we unpegged three towels, placed them on the concrete and cuddled up to each other as best we could, using our rucksacks for pillows.

PART IX

We shake hands and hug Louise's family, all down from Scotland. Catch up briefly with the last year or so. And then the hearse comes around the corner and we stand to the side. And it drives right through our small talk. I look to the floor, catch a glimpse of tears and a tiny coffin. Into the crematorium we shuffle, picking up the order of service that Richard made. A picture of tiny fingers being held by Mummy. Name tag around wrist.

Sophie Elizabeth Peace - born asleep, 26th July 2009

I contain myself while tears flow around me. I have to. And then, after prayers, I walk forwards, turn around and read out the poem I've been asked to. Back next to Anna, I allow myself to shake and cry, my natural feelings to find their way through. And then it's finished, and after hugs and tears and handshakes everyone has left except Anna, Matt and myself.

"It seemed so short," I say.

"Fifteen minutes," says Matt, shrugging.

We walk over to bunches and wreaths of flowers, read messages from Granny and Grandad, Mummy and Daddy. And we cry in unison at how unfair it is.

"I don't believe in God," says Anna.

"Neither do I," I say.

And then slowly up the lane in silence we walk, until another hearse comes around the corner, forcing us to stand to the side and bow our heads. A gathering of people follow it, carrying a coffin made of wicker. Nobody wears black, in stark contrast to ourselves and everyone that was in this lane just minutes ago. Bright colours with heads up. A homemade sign held aloft with cards pinned to it. The celebration of a life lived, rather than the mourning and emptiness of a life not started outside the womb.

Anna opened the door to our dingy bedsit, saw me kicking the oven, heard me swearing.

"Hey," she shouted. "What's up?"

I turned around, picked up my bottle of Newcastle Brown Ale, took a swig.

"I can't do this fucking cooking lark"

Turned back again and kicked the oven.

She put her bag on the bed, turned the gas down, glanced at the empty bottles sticking out the bin. Opened the door to our tiny oven, checked the sausages.

"They're fine. What are you getting so stressed for?"

I slumped on the bed and sighed.

The bedsit was in Gloucester Place, parallel to Baker Street, London W1. A three-quarter size bed took up half the space. Above, a tiny window that refused to open looked out onto rooftops. Outside, a shared toilet and shower that fused the electricity, meaning you had to run down four flights of stairs with a towel wrapped round you and shampoo dribbling in your eyes to switch it back on again. And there was no fire escape. The building was owned by The Duke of Devonshire but he wouldn't have spat in it. Wouldn't have lowered himself to even set foot in it.

Anna stuck a fork in potatoes now simmering gently.

"What was work like?"

"Same as usual"

"Right, well. We need to go to the launderette tonight"

We moved to the bedsit for two reasons. Firstly because my friends we'd initially moved in with after arriving in London had broken their relationship. And secondly because we intended saving money to travel to the Far East. To India. Perhaps Thailand and Vietnam. Three months later we had the total sum of no pounds whatsoever. I worked in Topman, Oxford Circus, half heartedly trying to sell Wrangler Jeans to tourists who wanted Levis. Anna was on the home care in Clapham. At first, having our own place was exciting. And it was summer too. I walked back from work through Regent's Park, waited for Anna under the same tree each night. On the weekend we wandered by the canal to Camden, listened to music, browsed second hand clothes and bookshops. But Anna grew up in the Peak District, found London constricting. The only people she knew were close friends of mine and though they were welcoming, she felt like an attachment. Our relationship suffered. Our life became claustrophobic. The future we'd dreamed about moved further away from us. We lost sight of each other amongst the polluted streams of dirty traffic. The sharp elbows of a life too busy.

The first student to walk into my class tells me another prisoner has hung himself, was found dead in his cell just hours ago. I'm not surprised when he tells me the name, but I am saddened. Alan was thirty-three but would have been sixty before he was released. He left my creative writing class three months ago. Left all education at the same time. I last saw him two weeks ago, on my way to the wing when he shouted down the corridor.

"Richard..."

I turned around and smiled, the first time I'd seen him in months.

"I've just finished your book mate, its mint. I got it from the library, really enjoyed it"

"Thank you"

"I've been away for a bit 'cause my head's not been right. But I'm getting myself sorted now, getting back into education. I'm signing up for creative writing again so I'll see you there"

I was pleased and told him so. I also told him he was a very good writer, had a talent for it. But I knew he'd tried to hang himself a couple of times in the last few months. That he had a serious drug problem and twenty-seven more years inside. He'd talked about it during class. How difficult it was to keep his motivation raised. How easy it was to carry on taking heroin instead.

The prisoners talk about him a few minutes. Then I bring their minds back to today, tell them we're playing a game on the five senses. I ask them to hear music that means something, give them a few moments, then go round one by one. The first says he heard rock music, was at a live gig. Another heard "joyous" classical music his mother used to play. I ask them to smell flowers. One smells marigolds, pictures himself walking through a poly tunnel full of them. "I'm walking right through the smell," he says, closing his eyes. Another smells the chrysanthemums downstairs in the yard, says he's been locked up so long he can't imagine smelling any others. They see different types of fish, a goldfish at a grandmother's house, a pike in a pond, mackerel on the end of fishing line. They feel soft sand, wet sand and builders' sand, taste salt on fish and chips, on roasted peanuts and on wind whipping up from waves onto a sailing boat that dips and rises out to sea. Then all is quiet and reflective. And I'm about to talk about how powerful the senses are, how they take us on journeys, when suddenly the rain comes lashing down outside. So we go to the windows and stand transfixed by its power.

"I walk slower in the rain," says one.

I look across and two of the other prisoners are nodding their heads.

"The officers don't understand. They think I'm taking the piss, or that I don't want to go to education. But it's not that. I just want to spend a few more seconds in the outside, a few more seconds feeling alive"

"Look at those swallows," says another, pointing.

"There's three of them"

We watch them swoop and dive over the yard, surrounded by walls of brick, tiny cell windows embedded every few yards, some with milk bottles balanced precariously on outside ledges. They dive and dance in the pouring rain, free and carefree, oblivious to enchanted eyes that watch from behind barred windows.

"I see them out my window," says one, then points over D-Wing. "See the top of those trees over there? My cell window looks out that way"

The others look envious.

"I can see the top half of the trees over the perimeter wall. It took me four and a half years to get that cell. I watch them playing there"

The swallows land on wire that covers all open spaces. That is lined with brightly coloured balls to act as a deterrent against helicopters. And then the rain stops as suddenly as it started and the clouds break apart to allow fractions of sunlight. And the prisoner who smelled the chrysanthemums leans forward and looks down at them in the yard.

"Is it just me or are those flowers even brighter than normal?"

I look down and he's right. They're resplendent, vibrant. As intense as the energy that fills the room.

"I slow down to smell the flowers as well," he says. "My ambition is to walk across the edge of the grass one day. Just a few yards. Just to be able to feel it under my feet"

There's a small moment of contemplation when the suicide of Alan is mentioned in the staff room. I imagine his last moments on earth, how he must have looked to the prison officer that found him. Then I drive home, put on a CD I picked up this morning, one I haven't played in about ten years. I skip through songs. None of them feel right. But then I settle on number five, and it fits:

Embrace the wind with both arms / Stop the clouds in the sky / Hang your head no more / And beg no more / Brother Wolf and Sister Moon / Your time has come

I turn the CD off when the song finishes, drive the rest of the way home in silence. When I get back to my street I pass five or six young men in suits, heading down to the main road, carnations in button holes.

I couldn't look at her when the van came. It parked outside and this bloke called Steve knocked on the door. I opened it, couldn't look him in the eye either. We'd made our best shot of it, done a runner from the Duke of Devonshire. Moved in with good friends in Camberwell. Saving money was impossible, so we'd decided to try and save our relationship instead. But living with friends just diluted our time together. Papered over cracks that ran through our relationship like valleys from another era. The hedonistic fun and discovery I'd encountered when first moving to London had been blown away by the world opening its borders to me. And the tight knotted group of friends I'd made were beginning to naturally splinter. Camberwell was just another place in London and London was depressing. Life was a slog that produced no results and no sense of optimism that things would pick up anytime, while the joy and adventure our relationship had been built on was stifled. We had no money to rekindle adventure and so looked elsewhere instead.

I pleaded for it to be me that left but Anna insisted, wouldn't have it any other way. These were my friends she said, even though they'd grown to love her too. She found a place after two weeks of trying. After two weeks of trying to pretend we were dealing with everything okay, as rational adults. Two weeks of sleeping in the same bed and being afraid to touch each other. Of not being able to look each other in the eye and not being able to talk with friends unless the other was out getting drunk. Then she found a room in Borough. Was going to share a ground floor flat with someone called Steve and his brother who had a number of aliases.

Jonny and Debs started lifting boxes. I couldn't just stand there so I helped too. It didn't take long. She hadn't enough time to collect much. And then we had a hug that wasn't a hug. Just a quick touching with heads turned aside. Jonny and Debs gave her real hugs, fought back tears for our sakes. And then she walked off with this bloke called Steve. Climbed into his van and drove away.

Anna wakes with an overwhelming sadness she's unable to shake off. When the day starts properly, when things need doing, when children swing into action, demand attention, then she'll be the usual Mammy. Getting things organised, sorting out feuds. Taking time to cuddle and smile, encourage and praise. But it has lain with her all night this sadness, its sticky closeness keeping her awake. Sinking and mixing with medication. She opens her eyes. I rub her head softly, her half a centimetre of dark brown hair starting to give good covering.

"It's all soft," I say.

She tries to smile, but not too hard. This new growth was supposed to symbolise something else, arrive in this world alongside her.

I walked down Streatham High Road, the capital's busiest, accustomed to fumes and noise that pervaded every pore. That stuttered through the traffic clogged streets of London, down every side street and back alley. It wasn't set to be the most exciting New Year's Eve. Anna and Debs were holed up with flu in a small Brixton Hill flat. But I wasn't hoping for partying. I was after something much more memorable and longer lasting. They sat in their 'living room', a tiny box with cushions on the floor and a telly in the corner. We had a smoke and a drink, watched telly. Midnight garnered a smile, then the girls decided to head for bed. As had been the case for the last six months I slept in Anna's bedroom, on the far side of her double mattress. It was where I belonged on those rare times we spent a night under the same roof. Neither of us questioned it. We hadn't seen each other for six months after the split. Couldn't put ourselves under such emotional pressure. Then we spent six months becoming nothing more than good friends. But by the end of 1998 I'd decided we were soul mates after all. I walked into Anna's bedroom and it wasn't just Anna that was right, it was everything around her too. Her style and balance reflected in the space. Her ornaments and posters. Her way of turning a drab room into a romantic Arabian boudoir. How she accomplished perfect feng shui with no money and no know-how. She lay on her side facing the middle of the room. Facing away from the unoccupied side of the bed I would slip into. Smiled as I walked over, took a sip of her herbal tea. I noticed her arms, her neck, her shoulders as she stretched to collect the alarm clock, make sure it was turned off. I wanted to kiss them, wanted to slide myself on top of her. More than anything, I wanted to hold her properly, like we used to. Clinging onto each other whilst everything else crumbled all around us. It was all we had once, all we needed. I walked round to the other side of the bed, sat down gently. Started to take my trousers off. Two people facing different directions but with an energy that pulled us together. An energy that had diminished but never died and now grew stronger than ever. Perhaps alcohol would have dissolved that increased awareness of energy, allowed actions more instantaneous. But alcohol wasn't the drug of our choice back then. Stoned, the energy became all, became everything, dragged our muscles and fibres. But with it came paranoia that this energy existed solely within our own minds. It sat on our shoulders, this paranoia. Sliced doubts into us. I pulled trousers off my ankles, jumper over my head. Threw them in a heap. The boxer shorts stayed on, the t-shirt too.

Anna spoke quietly without turning round, a hint of crackle in her soft voice.

"Can I turn the light off now?"

"Yeah...of course you can"

She laid down facing that way. And I laid down facing the other. And neither of us slept because we were so focused on what was behind us. And though eventually we must have drifted off to sleep, the energy didn't turn itself off, never had done. It charged across the cold section of bed and connected us.

It's one of those days when you're pleased you weren't frightened by another wrong weather forecast. Where the ratio between blue sky and cloud is perfect, the variation in cloud too. Elongated spaceships and cotton wool balls tinged with fire edges. The wind buffets our hair, brings salty wet spray. Every so often the boat tips a little further and a wave crashes over. Soaks someone to the sound of laughter. Anna has a new wig, a shorter version. The longer one rubbed on clothes, became worn down. Ended up like split ends in desperate need of attention. This one's redder, looks great, though she wears it up much of the time so it doesn't rub. Right now it has a hat stamped firmly on top of it. The last thing you want when you're on a boat in the North Sea is for your wig to fly off in front of people you've never met. We pass Longstone Lighthouse, home of Grace Darling, who rescued nine men from the storm wrecked SS Forfarshire in 1838. Past rocks crusted in barnacles, embraced by seaweed, whitewashed with bird droppings. Seagulls following in the ridiculous notion that this is still a fishing boat that does what it was built for. Our weathered captain points out the burial place and church of St Cuthbert. There are over five hundred known shipwrecks around the Farne Islands, he tells us. They share this tiny part of the North Sea with cormorants, shags, kittiwakes and guillemots. With a colony of four thousand seals and seventy thousand puffins that arrive in spring to have their young. Coming here reminds Anna and I of our childhoods. I reach across, ruffle Joe's hair and smile. He doesn't move, just stares over the side at the glassy sea, looking for fish, wondering about crabs and lobsters. Stretching out to touch and dip fingers. We pass another family of seals, bobbing about in the sea, as curious about us as we are about them. Way back; Bamburgh Castle is visible on the mainland, imposing upon its rocky basalt crag. The royal seat of the ancient Kings of Northumbria. And further behind; the cheviots stretching high and wide into clouds. We jump out onto one of the islands with the help of the captain. Pick shells and take pictures of lazy seals. Then it's back into the boat again, all four families, including one from Japan, two older couples and two dogs. I stand as we roll and lurch. Shift weight from one leg to the other. Take sunshine and sea breeze into my face. Isla closes her eyes and rests her head on her Mammy's lap, her body wrapped in waterproofs. Joe rests the side of his head on his arms, continues staring out to sea, has never been so peaceful in waking moments. I wonder what he's thinking, looking out to sea like an old fisherman with so many regrets, so many memories. We come back past Inner Farne, its 14ᵗʰ century chapel on the site where St Cuthbert lived from 676 to 684. Before he was allowed to live on the island he promised to banish 'demons' from there. Later inhabitants occasionally caught sight of them though, described them as "clad in cowls, riding upon goats, black in complexion, short in stature, their countenances most hideous, their heads long." It's thought these demons were descendants of early settlers or `aborigines' who had been cut off from the mainland. And now this mainland comes closer, the pier appearing to drift across water towards us. I look across at Anna, Isla still sleeping on her lap. Her eyes seem wistful and far away, remembering those holidays with her family, her brother peering over the edge like her son now. We're half an hour later than we should be. The captain was enjoying himself too much, the passengers too peaceful and contemplative. Past the pier we go, past families fishing, lobster pots and floating gulls. Anna wakes her daughter with a kiss. The boat is docked perfectly and we're the last to get off. Joe needs a nudge into action. Anna looks across at me.

"That was beautiful," she says. "I feel quite emotional, like I'm about to cry"

"I know," I say. "I could tell. And anyway, so do I"

I brought early morning tea, watched her bare arms as she stretched, raised herself on elbow to drink. Then I sat on the bottom of the bed, on her side this time, watched as she took her first sip.

"Well. It's 1999"

She smiled, said nothing. Always was a little sleepy first thing in the morning.

"What are you hoping for?"

She took another sip while she pondered the question.

"What? From 1999?"

"Yeah. What are you hoping for this year?"

She shrugged, as if it were a stupid question.

"I'm just hoping for a better year than the last one"

I smiled. And we both looked down.

But after five seconds of silence I reinstated my topic.

"I'd like this year to be the start of something"

Her eyes met mine, inquisitive.

"Would you?"

"Yeah, or maybe I should say the re-start of something"

And this time our eye contact held.

"I want it to be the re-start of us Anna. I miss you"

She looked like she was going to cry. I touched her on the knee, the duvet between us. The most important decision of my life was in front of me, but it wasn't mine to take.

"I didn't know what I had until I lost you. I want you back darling"

She said nothing. Maybe I'd stunned her. Perhaps she'd

started seeing someone else. I started to get nervous, began to plead.

"I have no doubt in my mind whatsoever that I want to be with you, for the rest of my life. I love you and I think we belong together. I know we do"

Still nothing...

"I haven't just come to this decision all of a sudden you know. I've been thinking it over for months, making sure it was the right one. I needed to know within myself that if I asked you out again it would be forever. And it is. I don't want to go through that break up again. I don't want you to go through it either. It was horrible. But I haven't been the same without you. And I know now that I love you and I want to be with you again...I won't let you down...I promise"

She took her eyes away from mine for the first time, looked to the wall.

"What are you thinking? Speak to me"

"I don't know," she said. "I don't know if I can put myself through it all again"

"Put yourself through what? I want this for good. I want you forever. If you want me then there's no risk"

"I can't make my mind up, not just like that"

"So you're not giving me an answer then?"

She pulled the duvet tighter round her knees.

"No," she said. "I'm not. I need to think about it"

I walk up to Anna and rub her hair.

"It's like a long haired tennis ball"

She looks up.

"Are you taking the micky out of me?"

"Of course I'm not. It's lovely"

And so she smiles, another one of those half smiles.

"It's eyelashes and eyebrows I'm after. I didn't mind my head being bald. I got used to that"

I look at her face while she checks my eyes for giveaway signs and I try not to show any. She may look a little odd without eyelashes and eyebrows. But her face has serene beauty, aided by steroids that can puff faces up, but in a slim face like Anna's simply irons out thirty-something motherhood lines. She has the movements and aura of someone who has found peace before death. That beautiful stillness before the first crack of lightning. I'm hoping those dark clouds will be pushed away by the winds that come over the North Sea. That chinks of light will open up into bright sunshine once more. But Anna says she would feel like this forever if it allowed Sophie Elizabeth to have lived.

I ask how her chest is, now she's nearly finished radiotherapy.

She pulls her top open. It blushes red.

"It's peeling," she says, "like sunburn. It's sore like sunburn as well"

Then she tells me she saw her boss today, says he's sympathetic but doesn't understand. Couldn't possibly know what it's like for her. He did agree to a staggered return though, and her working the same days as before.

"How would you sum it up then?" I ask.

"I was just pleased to get my point across and not burst into tears," she answers.

It comes in a plain white envelope. There's no urgency when I open it. I presume it's just usual junk mail. But then I pull it from the ripped envelope and see the publisher's logo on top, notice the first sentence: I enclose our new form of royalty statement for your book published by us. I'm aware there's a second page behind but I continue to read, saving the best part for last. This statement summarises all incomes on your book. I've already e-mailed a couple of times asking how many books I've sold but I've not had any response yet so I'm caught completely off guard. I turn to the second page. UK & Commonwealth Sales (paperback) - £439.82. There's a list below that but dashes rather than numbers are the order of the day. I skip to the bottom, past advances paid to date and returns provision, and my eyes settle on Total £170.13. I smile, walk over, hand both pages to Anna, sitting on the couch with Isla watching Peppa Pig. Three years hard work and the dreams of many more. I imagined debates on Radio 4, walking through revolving doors as tall as a giant but dressed better. I dreamt I would turn into someone with an aura about them. Someone who had written something that had an impact. But I'm subbing off someone who's been on the sick for nine months, pretending that everything will be okay. That I'll get a couple of grand at the least, pay off my credit card. Either that or lift me out of my overdraft, provide some leeway for a few months. But instead of all this, I'm getting £170. Anna reacts as calmly as she ever does, but still manages to mutter "bloody hell" under her breath. I walk away thinking 'I got the car serviced last week, it cost over £400.' Anna comes over, says she's sorry, starts to pull my head towards her chest. I pull away, hate anyone feeling pity for me.

"There's your new kitchen," I say.

She smiles.

"Maybe we'll just get a new pepper grinder instead"

So Anna tidies our shabby kitchen and gets used to the fact it's staying with us longer than she hoped for. I get Joe from Nippers, read him a book in bed and look on the bright side. Come down as Anna's finishing.

"Well, at least I can say I got seven hundred quid"

She looks surprised.

"What?"

"At least I can say I got seven hundred quid. One hundred and seventy plus five hundred advance. That's nearly seven hundred"

Now she looks confused.

"You mean you don't owe them?"

"What?"

"Maybe I read the statement wrong," she says.

I go and get it, show her where it says total £170.13.

She runs her finger down the line of numbers, adds my five hundred advance to returns of £109.96, takes that away from royalties of £439.82 and then points at the tiny dash that I hadn't noticed before the £ sign.

"That's a minus darling. You owe them £170 pounds"

Smiles apologetically.

I've got my trainers tied up within two minutes. Within

ten I'm on the beach walking Caffrey. Wind pushes the tide into peaks that arc and crash on rocks as white as swirling cream. A man throws stones into the sea for his dog while his girlfriend takes pictures of fire clouds. I march on, step over dozens of washed up jellyfish. Walk all the way to Blyth with fists clenched.

Sleet hammered off the roof, blinded our way. Sent windscreen wipers into manic mode as we crawled along ever slower.

"We're not going to make it," said Anna. "It's getting worse"

"We could stop overnight at your Mam's," said my cousin Martin, who needed some relief after driving for six hours.

And so, after a warm family welcome in Hartlepool, we woke to beautiful sunshine and continued up the North-East coast. Past Newcastle to a place called Seaton Sluice. A month before we'd never heard of the place. But we knew we needed to get away from London. Another year together had told us that. We wanted to live by the sea but be in touch with a city. Newcastle was the obvious choice. Anna had studied there. My family were under forty miles away and Anna's family had spent summer holidays on the coast of Northumberland. We took a week off, went to stay with my parents. Caught the train to Newcastle, the metro to Whitley Bay. The first five estate agents refused to deal with us. We had no savings, might not get benefits because we'd be leaving jobs voluntarily, were both credit black listed. But then we turned up at a small place called

Property Quarters, met a woman called Mandy. She liked us, said she trusted us, would help us find a place, though Whitley Bay and Tynemouth were far too expensive.

"How about Seaton Sluice?" she asked. "Would you live there? We've got a house for rent there"

"I've never heard of it. Is it near the sea?"

She smiled.

"Let's get in my car. I'll drive you up there to have a look"

So off we went with this woman we'd just met, who we would see just once more in our lives, passing in a supermarket years later. A woman who would never know just how important she was to our lives. A few miles north of Whitley Bay, in between there and Blyth. She showed us a small terraced house, took us along the seafront just down the road. We looked out the windscreen at sand dunes, at the beach. At a little harbour full of fishing boats. And we fell in love. We didn't know then that Seaton Sluice, or Hartley as it was known in the 19th century, was once a bustling sea port with brigs, barques and sloops trading cargoes of salt, coal, bottle, glass and copperas to London, southern England and the continent. We didn't know it employed hundreds of seamen, provided a living for miners, rope makers, sail makers, shipbuilders and many other professions. That it had the largest bottle works in the country. Nor did we know that attempts were made to turn it into a popular seaside resort once its industrial life ended in 1871 with the closure of the bottleworks. A railway line was eventually built for such a purpose. But then the Great War broke out and the tracks were removed to use elsewhere. All we saw was a sleepy seaside village far away from inner city London. We fell in love with its solitude and signed the forms as soon as we were back in the office. We couldn't remember anything whatsoever about the house when my Dad asked later that day, but it didn't matter. The next morning we got the train to Newcastle again, jumped the metro to Whitley Bay. Walked to Seaton Sluice along sand, rocks and cliff. Hand in hand the whole way.

People ask when Anna will find out if she has the all clear. I tell them it's presumed she has already, that she doesn't have cancer anymore. The lumpectomy, mastectomy, chemotherapy, radiotherapy and Tamoxifen were like five big sledgehammers to crack a little cluster of wicked nuts. But their questions gnaw at me, make me realise I've been so consumed by the present I've only presumed about the long term future. Either that or I simply haven't dared to delve too deeply. And so I ask Anna when the kids are in bed. She says there's a fifteen per cent chance of secondary's, of the cancer returning within the next five years. If that happens then it won't be curable. It will be a case of managing it as best as she can for as long as she can until it finally kills her. I don't know what to say. Anna looks at me like it's something she's always known. Shrugs.

I have to do a double take when I see her on the computer. She doesn't have the time or inclination usually. So I wander across, peer over her shoulder.

"It's my sleeping," she says. "I'm so tired. I'm only getting one and a half, two hours sleep. Then I'm awake the rest of the night"

"I know darling"

She scrolls down messages.

"There's hundreds of people here all with the same problem, all with Tamoxifen. Exactly the same. They sleep the first couple of hours then that's it"

She looks across at me but her eyes are working backwards, considering for a moment.

"It says here thirty-six percent of people end up coming off Tamoxifen"

"How long have you got left on it?"

"Two and a half years," she says. "Then two and a half years on another drug. Either that or all five on Tamoxifen. I don't think I can go that long without sleeping"

Martin pulled up outside our small terraced house. We dumped boxes inside, said hello to two giant Newfoundland dogs that wandered in to have a look. Took the picnic my Mam made and went to explore. Martin was just as excited as we were and it was appropriate that he drove us to our new life; the son of my Daddy's brother who moved to Australia before I was born. He and his partner Corinna had stayed with us in our Brixton Hill flat for six months, moved out just before we left. The three of us explored the fishing harbour, the cliffs above Charlie's Garden. We went down the steep path to Collywell Bay, climbed rocks and threw stones in the sea. We ate our sandwiches on a flat section halfway up a cliff, now immortalised as Martin's Picnic Spot. On the night we went for a pub crawl, ran down the beach under dazzling stars towards the fifth. Stopped to look out into darkness and the sound of waves. There's something about the coast, about being on the edge of land, looking off into a horizon of sea. It places you somewhere in the world, on a wider scale. It gives perspective to greater life. When I lived in Brixton Hill I used to lie awake at night pretending the constant traffic was the sound of waves. Now the waves were about the same distance away. And I knew then, that whenever we were in need of solace or healing, of inner balance, the waves would be there for us with their constant movement and sway to the moon's tide.

It's the night before Anna's due back at work. She's in the kitchen waiting for the kettle to boil. I walk up, ask if she's okay. All of a sudden she looks worse than before, as if my question flicked a switch.

"I get really anxious," she says, putting a hand to her chest.

I walk up, cuddle her, step back to listen.

"I know it's stupid. And I know it will probably be fine. But I've been in my safety bubble for so long"

"But you have been going out," I say. "You haven't stopped in the house for the last six months have you? You've seen lots of people, been loads of places"

"I know. But it's with people I know, in places I'm comfortable"

The water bubbles and boils. She picks the kettle up, looks back at me.

"I don't want to be amongst a crowd. I don't think I could handle it"

"Mmmm...I don't suppose the childcare problem will help either"

"No," she says. "It's the last thing I need. And I don't know if my anxiousness is because of cancer or because of that. Or just a symptom of the Tamoxifen and chemo"

Her boss has gone back on his word, of her working the same days as before, despite it meaning we'd have to pay for childcare five days each week but only use it for two changing ones. You signed your flexible working contract he said yesterday, when she phoned him up and received her timetable. Anna's worried because she knows the council are looking to make redundancies, thinks maybe it's a way of bringing things to a head.

I sat on the wall waiting, my guts tightening at how much impact the next half hour could have on our lives. Looking across the square for what seemed like the hundredth time, I tapped the heel of my shoe, flaked cement that spun onto the ground below. Anna was late. One of the most important moments in our lives. Two years of trying and failing. Of tests in hospitals and the Centre for Life. And there we were at the end of the process, about to receive results for both of us. Find out if one of us was infertile. And she couldn't even get there in time.

When I saw her come round the corner I jumped off the wall.

"Where the hell have you been?"

She produced it from her pocket, this little white stick.

"What's that?"

"A pregnancy test"

Unbeknown to me, she'd decided to do a pregnancy test in the toilets in Whitley Bay metro station. She didn't hold out much hope but she'd had PMT for over a week so decided to try just in case. And there she was, holding this stick out in front of me, her mouth starting to curl upwards into a smile of disbelief.

"What does it say?" I asked. "What's the result?"

"It's positive," she smiled.

"What?"

"It's positive darling. I'm pregnant"

I scratched my head.

"Are you sure?"

She laughed.

"Yes I'm sure. I got it out three times on the metro to check"

The door goes. I cheer. Isla looks round in expectation. She's earlier than we thought she'd be, in time for tea. We walk to the kitchen door, look across. See her putting her bag down, taking her coat off. She's smiling, looks as normal as can be. And for a second or two it's like the previous ten months never happened. Like she never had eight and a half months off work. Never had cancer. Never had a mastectomy, chemotherapy, any of that. Isla screams in delight, runs across to her Mammy, grabs her leg. I wait in the kitchen and smile, hug her when she comes my way, flick the kettle on.

She took hold of my shoulders and shook.

"What?"

"It's my contractions. I'm having them"

"Mmmm...what's the time between them?"

I'd been to antenatal classes, knew what questions to ask.

"They're coming every four to five minutes"

But I was sleepy. I thought she said forty-five minutes. So I snuggled back to dreamland.

She woke me at seven, said I'd better take Caffrey for a quick walk, she needed to go in. By eight a.m. we were parked at North Tyneside General Hospital and Anna was afraid to take her hands off the roof of the car because her contractions were coming one after the other. We were sent straight to delivery. She was nine centimetres dilated. Her plan of having every pain killer possible was shelved. It was too late for any of them. An hour later they took the gas and air from her too. Then at 11.32 a.m., on Monday 30ᵗʰ June 2003, Anna gave birth to a baby boy weighing six pounds and nine ounces. He cried at the shock of it all, while Anna's head fell back on the pillow. But within a few seconds he'd latched firmly onto her full breast.

I stumble out the house at seven a.m., the first day of 2010. Amazed at the sight of so much snow piling around me. Four or five inches already, blanketing everything, none of which had been present when I'd gone to bed six hours earlier. I walk down the street towards the cliffs. Excited at making the first footprints of the New Year but aware they'll be covered again soon. And then, wrapped up warm, snowflakes glistening around my face, clinging to the fake fur of my snorkel hood, I appear on the edge of the cliff, look at the grey sea and grey sky. Snow falling everywhere like the distorted picture on a television screen. I walk along the edge, struck at how I could be anywhere. Antarctica, Alaska, the inhospitable Siberian tundra. Beach and rocks frozen white. The sea as far out as the moon can drag it. I notice a tiny spot of red down below on the beach, shift my hood back and place a gloved hand above my head to stop the falling snow impeding my view. A man hunches over a bucket, digging for worms. And then I turn to the path again, to where it continues, further from the houses, towards the sea. And as I walk under snow that falls even heavier I see a woman coming the other way. Her dog runs up to Caffrey and they fall about in the snow together. Then the woman and I are close. And our eyes meet, glistening under hats and hoods, a connection that needs no words. An experience shared by just the two of us.

"What a way to start the New Year," I say.

She smiles and points back to where she came from, where I am headed, further out to sea.

"When you get out there," she says, "it's all one, and you're in the centre of it"

"Good," I smile back. "That's what I want. That's why I'm out here"

And she waves me off as I carry on forwards...

Joe was a long thin baby with chicken legs and an insatiable appetite. For the first three months of his life he was an almost constant attachment to Anna's breasts. He slept for an hour or so, then woke up starving. Anna would roll over, pick him up, remove her breast pad and clamp him on. For the first few weeks I would wake up every time too, watch in sleepy amazement over the beautiful curve of Anna's breast. Joe, with wide open eyes, glugging away fast and noisily as if his whole life depended upon it. And it did, it really did. When he'd managed to fill most of his ravenous hunger he would relax and slow down, make slow sucking noises of contentment. Purr like a cat that got plenty of cream. Then his eyes would become heavier and heavier until he eventually drifted back off into contented slumber.

I got the phone call at work. Anna was having pains at playgroup. I needed to go home. Half an hour later we were off to North Tyneside General again, leaving Joe with Anna's Mum. And at 4.35p.m., on Friday March 10th 2006, Anna gave birth for the second time. Laid back and smiled.

"I've given you the baby girl you wanted to go with your boy," she said.

I cried and went to phone our families. And Isla came into our lives, a dark haired baby, placid and easy to manage, content when she got older to simply sit on her bum and watch her older brother run about.

PART X

We wake to the roar of waves rather than the sweet melody of birdsong. The Atlantic Ocean meets the Mediterranean Sea and crashes just beneath our balcony, as it has done all night, sending torrents of foam and spray surging into the sky. The girls are in the bathroom, are not allowed to come out. Anna's in the bath, doing Isla's nails at the same time. Joe and I are putting suits on, checking ourselves out in the full length mirror. Choosing flip-flops because our trainers were soaked through in yesterday's downpour and we didn't have enough space in the suitcases to bring shoes. Then we're out. But not before insisting the girls keep the bathroom door shut so they can't see us go past. And two minutes later we're back again anyway. I forgot the umbrella. And so we miss the bus by seconds, ask the receptionist to order a taxi instead, stand outside the hotel and watch barbary apes roll over and play fight, chase each other along the wall, leap onto customers cars.

Half an hour later we're button-holed, flip-flopping through the streets of Gibraltar. I'm pulling Joe by the hand because the first florist was closed and the second, when we eventually found it, didn't have any fresh flowers. And so I'm pulling Joe by one hand and carrying a bouquet of orange chrysanthemums in the other and we're dashing and weaving through streets filling with slow moving shoppers and too relaxed tourists. I yank Joe onto the pavement to stop him crashing into an elderly couple, again when a car comes slowly rolling through. People glance at our suits, our carnations, understand, smile in admiration. Then their eyes move downwards towards our flip-flops and the lines in the middle of their foreheads crinkle. I want to explain we expected hot sunshine this far south in spring. But we don't have time. I look upwards instead, towards darkening grey clouds, pray the rain will hold off a couple of hours, that it won't pour down on us with as much power as it did yesterday. Please. Not for this. We flip-flop through the gates with a minute to spare, arrive with an apology that the bride had to wait for the bridegroom instead of the other way round. Anna looks beautiful, her hair now shoulder length, layered and shining. Her dark red wedding dress clinging to her fantastic figure. Cupping two beautiful breasts, one an expert reconstruction. Hugging her waist and bottom before billowing out stylishly to the ground. Isla has a red dress on too, ruffled around the neck, looks gorgeous. The boys compliment the girls. The girls compliment the boys. And then the registrar turns up, with his gentle demeanour and eyes full of love. He explains the process, meets the two witnesses Anna found twenty minutes earlier; a gardener and the official photographer I'd booked the week before.

He asks us to recite our vows. We look into each other's eyes and smile. Say them clearly. Isla looks on with curiosity as Joe hands out wedding rings. We kiss, pose for photographs, kiss again. Happy as we ever could be, once more. And then the sun comes out to shine its warmth upon us as we wander around winding paths and the Mediterranean flora of these beautiful Botanical Gardens.

Standing in a queue, waiting for the cable car. The woman in the kiosk notices our outfits, asks if we've just been married, lets the children on for free. Then boxed in tight with another dozen people, we rise through the air, look down at the marina, patient freighters, the runway that extends into the sea, that dissects this Monolithic rock, one of the pillars of Hercules, from the mainland of Spain.

Isla takes her hands away from the window, faces me.

"I'm hungry Daddy"

"I'm not surprised," I tell her. "We paid ten pounds for your breakfast this morning and all you had was two slices of ham"

She grins, turns back to the window, the view beyond. Joins Joe in his speechless fascination at rising through the air.

Then we're outside, right on top. And the clouds are drifting down to meet us, tightening into heavy dank gloom that causes tourists to curl shoulders and zip up tight. The apes don't care about the weather. They delight everyone by strolling around nonchalantly, posing for photographs on the very edge, leaping about when the urge takes them. One tries to grab Anna's bouquet of chrysanthemums but she holds on tight. It grabs a few petals instead, puts them to its mouth. Spits them out when it finds they're not tasty. The clouds tighten further until there's nothing to be seen except grey. And then the rain starts, light at first but within ten seconds it's flooding down, drenching us. It doesn't matter though, not anymore. Nature will take its course, will throw whatever it wants at us. We accept whatever it gives, will always appreciate our time together now, don't need to remind ourselves of the important things in life. I had a dream last night that I stepped off the edge of a high dusty cliff. But I didn't fall. I floated...

Anna takes refuge in the visitors centre, takes the kids with her. Rainwater soaks into my jacket and trousers, dampens my skin as I stare into grey. I was expecting to see Africa over there on the far horizon. I turn, watch Anna brush down her wedding dress, look out the window, Joe and Isla climbing up onto tall stools. Then I turn north and again see nothing but cloud and rain. But that doesn't matter either. I know what's on the other side. I'm able to drift through the damp and imagine the near future, to where train tracks wind their way through hills and valleys, through the gorges and whitewashed villages of Andalucía.

And then I turn back to Anna and she shrugs.

And smiles.

Author's Note

When Anna was diagnosed with breast cancer I wrote every day because it helped, and about our past in case it was all our children would be left with. Initially, there was no thought about turning this writing into a book; it was simply a way to help me cope. I believe creative writing has great therapeutic power and can act as a powerful tool for self-esteem and balance, as well as making fascinating reading that can inform and influence a wider public.

I currently teach creative writing at HMP Frankland and am editor of the prison magazine. Previously I have been Writer in Residence at HMP Durham and have helped facilitate three creative projects at HMP Low Newton. Some of the written work from these projects, as well as relevant artwork, can be found in the book, 'Shattered Images and Building Bridges,' also published by Lapwing Books. In the future, I plan to continue throughout society, helping others tell tales and write stories that are respected and hopefully admired by others - but most importantly by those that have written them.

I welcome comments and suggestions at:
richard.whardwick@yahoo.co.uk

You can find extracts, soundtracks, videos and much more at my website:
www.richardwhardwick.co.uk

Read occasional ramblings at my blog:
www.richardwhardwick.wordpress.com

Or perhaps find me lazing about on Facebook

Acknowledgements

Richard is currently writing his third book, the one that was going to be his second novel until a diagnosis in February 2009 interrupted his mind as well as the life of him and his family.

He would like to thank the following:

My Mam and Dad, otherwise known as Granny Annie and Grandad Barry

Anna's Mum and Dad, otherwise known as Building Granny and Building Grandad

Richard, Louise and Sophie Elizabeth

Rachael, Mike, Jasmine, Rosie and Lily

The fantastic staff at North Tyneside General Hospital, the Royal Victoria Infirmary and the Freeman Hospital in Newcastle upon Tyne

All our wonderful friends in Seaton Sluice

All those wonderful friends who, given the book's structure, weren't mentioned in Andalucía because of issues of timing or location

Anthony Nott for his support and editing advice, enabling me to shred those unnecessary pages

Thanks also:

Claire Tustin for that all important proof read

Dawn Felicia Lehrer, artist and friend, for allowing me to accompany her and write about the shop fitters in Sunderland that had closed down

Dave Harper, who first told me of Andalucía, and who played me the song of the same name by John Cale

Harry Palmer, Dawn and Dave for helping me understand that if I want to do something I should just go for it – and for providing such beautiful inspiration

Chris, Chloe and Charlie for helping me make the handmade Andalucia art books that I am giving away on my blog site

d_rradio for creating a musical interpretation of Andalucia, which I'm also planning to give away free

Alison, Suzy and Nicola at Durham City Arts - if only Governments fully understood the power of the arts and the role that agencies such as DCA and their employees play…

Lapwing Books is a micro-publisher and has no finance for marketing and publicity. We therefore respectfully request that if you enjoyed this book, you consider lending or recommending it to family, friend or colleague - or indeed buying it as a present for them.

With thanks